Diagnosis Narratives and the Healing Ritual in Western Medicine

W0113129

The dominance of "illness narratives" in narrative healing studies has tended to mean that the focus centers around the healing of the individual. Meza proposes that this emphasis is misplaced and the true focus of cultural healing should lie in managing the disruption of disease and death (cultural or biological) to the individual's relationship with society. By explicating narrative theory through the lens of cognitive anthropology, Meza reframes the epistemology of narrative and healing, moving it from relativism to a philosophical perspective of pragmatic realism. Using a novel combination of narrative theory and cognitive anthropology to represent the ethnographic data, Meza's ethnography is a valuable contribution in a field where ethnographic records related to medical clinical encounters are scarce. The book will be of interest to scholars of medical anthropology and those interested in narrative history and narrative medicine.

James P. Meza is Assistant Professor in the Department of Family Medicine and Public Health Science at Wayne State University School of Medicine, USA. He holds a PhD in Cultural Anthropology and is a practicing doctor of medicine (MD).

Routledge Studies in Health and Medical Anthropology

Depression in Kerala
Ayurveda and mental health care in 21st century India
Claudia Lang

Diagnosis Narratives and the Healing Ritual in Western Medicine
James P. Meza

www.routledge.com/Routledge-Studies-in-Health-and-Medical-Anthropology/
book-series/RSHMA

Diagnosis Narratives and the Healing Ritual in Western Medicine

James P. Meza

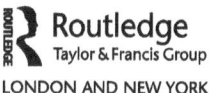

Routledge
Taylor & Francis Group

LONDON AND NEW YORK

First published 2019
by Routledge
2 Park Square, Milton Park, Abingdon, Oxon OX14 4RN

and by Routledge
52 Vanderbilt Avenue, New York, NY 10017, USA

First issued in paperback 2020

Routledge is an imprint of the Taylor & Francis Group, an informa business

British Library Cataloguing-in-Publication Data
A catalogue record for this book is available from the British Library

Library of Congress Cataloging-in-Publication Data
A catalog record for this book has been requested

ISBN 13: 978-0-367-58851-9 (pbk)
ISBN 13: 978-1-138-63142-7 (hbk)

Typeset in Sabon
by Apex CoVantage, LLC

Healing is the ritual process where a "self" facing annihilation by an existential threat navigates the liminal social space of alienation from the cultural body and reconnects with a new cultural role by forming a healing relationship with the socially authorized healer – the doctor.

Dedicated to K.A.C., who was there at the beginning of my journey of understanding and K.C.S., who encouraged me to write.

Contents

Figures

Preface

I always enjoy reading ethnographies. They are typically easy to read and help me understand what it is like to be in a different time or place – to understand how people live their lives differently than anything I had known before. The best ethnographies also have an important truth to reveal.

I am mindful of my reading audience. I wrote this book in the genre of ethnography capable of withstanding critique by any anthropologist. With the increasing awareness of the social determinants of health, I believe more doctors need to read ethnographies. A medical student who looked at an early draft manuscript told me he struggled with the theory but enjoyed the rest of the book. For medical readers, do not worry too much about theory and simply enjoy the book. Ethnography has helped me understand the social context of my own clinical practice in a way that nothing else can.

I also know that there are many doctors quite interested in narrative medicine (Brody 1994; Charon 2006; Elwyn and Gwyn 1999; Engel et al. 2008; Launer 2002). This book presents a unique perspective on narrative medicine. I hope physicians interested in narrative medicine can find a previously unrecognized description of their daily clinical practice.

For medical anthropologists interested in narrative healing, I recognize that this ethnography presents an iconoclastic perspective. Because anthropologists are more interested in theory than doctors are, I hope this book opens new theoretical perspectives. I hope to have pushed the field of narrative healing just a bit forward. I also think my synthetic theoretical discussion at the end of the book provides an opportunity to go back and question solidified attitudes while inviting further study.

By reaching a broad audience, I hope to have impact on medical education and health policy – unless we understand the core function of a doctor in society, we will continue to repeat our mistakes. American medicine is in turmoil and I hope getting back to basics has a clarifying effect. This is the gift anthropology offers. More than anything, I hope to instill how medicine and anthropology enhance each other by breaking down disciplinary barriers.

References

Brody, Howard. 1994. "My Story Is Broken; Can You Help Me Fix It?" Medical Ethics and the Joint Construction of Narrative. *Literature and Medicine* 33(1):79–92.

Charon, Rita. 2006. *Narrative Medicine Honoring the Stories of Illness.* Oxford: Oxford University Press.

Elwyn, Glyn, and Richard Gwyn. 1999. Narrative Based Medicine: Stories We Hear and Stories We Tell: Analysing Talk in Clinical Practice. *BMJ* 318(7177):186–188.

Engel, John D., et al. 2008. *Narrative in Health Care: Healing Patients, Practitioners, Profession, and Community.* Oxford: Radcliffe.

Launer, John. 2002. *Narrative-Based Primary Care.* Abingdon: Radcliffe Medical Press.

Acknowledgments

The American Academy of Family Physicians Foundation – Joint Grant Awards Program provided partial funding during data acquisition (G0907).

The Arnold P. Gold Foundation provided partial funding for data analysis (RS-15–005).

Part I
Methods

1   Fieldwork methods

Science is asking important questions; research is answering those questions. Anthropologists are scientists who explore, discover, understand, and describe culture. In this chapter, I report the intellectual and pragmatic components of how I accomplished those tasks for this research project.

Epistemology matters

Narrative theory is ubiquitous and informs many disciplines; it means different things to different people. The "self" is a highly contested construct. Living in a post-modern world, an in-depth reading of narrative and healing reveals a cacophony of opinions. To critically appraise this body of literature, I was advised to study philosophy because "it will help you think." I took the advice to heart (Cahoone 2010; Goldman 2006; Kasser 2006; Robinson 2004).

Qualitative writers often do not declare their epistemology, leaving the reader without a frame of reference to view claims by researchers (Cohen and Crabtree 2008). I believe that while we may never achieve a full understanding of reality, we can approximate it ever more closely through scientific endeavors. I adhere to an epistemological philosophy of pragmatic realism.[1] Bruno Latour opens his book with a challenge from another, "Do you believe in reality?" and answers, "But of course!" (Latour 1999). He was writing to extricate us from the "Science Wars" of post-modernism. Latour and I share a mutual epistemological perspective. Anthropological writing on healing in Western medicine relies predominantly on narrative theory, most often written from a relativist perspective. Although I can accept the value of contributions written from a relativist perspective, I believe they share only one perspective, leaving me the burden to integrate their work with that of others.

The seminal text that applied narrative theory to narrative healing was *The Illness Narratives: Suffering, Healing and the Human Condition* by Arthur Kleinman. Published in 1988, this text marked the beginning of "a narrative turn" in anthropological thought. With this text, the Harvard Friday Morning Narrative Group launched a landslide of narrative studies related to healing. Common to most all of these writings is an epistemological framework of relativism. Kleinman takes the semiotic nature of what people say about their illness as both a reflection of reality in medical practice as well as our cultural framework. Critiques of illness narratives point out that patients present themselves as social actors persuading themselves and the doctor to a potentially biased narrative, a form of relativism. Narrative and healing studies flourished, and Cheryl Mattingly and Linda Garro summarized the orthodox versions of narrative healing quite well (Mattingly and Garro 2000).

As a pragmatic realist, I am unwilling to accept everything written from a relativist perspective. While work written from that perspective contains partial truths, it remains incomplete and risks describing reified constructs. Phenomenological descriptions may not withstand the scientific imperative to replicate findings. My pragmatic realism resonates with the theoretical foundation of this ethnography.

Theory matters

Ethnography needs a theoretical foundation. My first task before starting fieldwork was to explicate my theoretical framework. Theory determines what questions can be asked, guides data collection, and organizes data for analysis. Because of prior training, I was initially attracted to psychoanalysis as a possible theoretical frame (Ewing 1990; Murphy and Murphy 2004). Yet, one of the primary reasons to do ethnography is to advance theory, and that is not possible with psychoanalysis – it only provides an organizing principle for ethnographic data. I next explored narrative theory because of the metonymically dominant phrase "narrative healing" in the anthropological canon. I was disillusioned with its relativism, something it shares with psychoanalysis (Rudnytsky and Charon 2008). Having confessed my dissatisfaction with relativist narrative theory, I used highly selective foundational theorists and generated an integrated theoretical frame for this work that combines narrative theory and cognitive anthropology. I present a rather parsimonious theoretical perspective that connects the vast body of anthropological work on healing to the current study while preserving my scientific pragmatism. I hope the reader appreciates how my ethnographic data and the theoretical frame I explicate support each other. For me, working with theory put a fresh perspective on narrative theory, which I had experienced as rather stale. I do not attempt to present a comprehensive review of narrative theory. This book is about healing, not narrative theory.

My favorite summary of narrative theory was written by Cheryl Mattingly (Mattingly 1998). If a reader wants a succinct summary of narrative theory, I recommend that text. I discuss theory to accomplish this research project because theory is part of the anthropological method of discovery.

The research question

The research question, "What is healing?" has occupied the past twenty years of my career. Physicians use the word "healing" often when reflecting on the practice of medicine, but there is no "meat on the bones" from a scientific perspective. Rather, when doctors talk about "healing," they usually appeal to the humanities.

Healing is a construct; it is not something observable under a microscope. I maintain that it *is* observable in cultural practices. The research question that guided this project was to clarify the domain analysis for "healing" to defend against the criticism that healing is a reified construct. For many years, I explored psychology, which claims to describe healing. I can only say that I exhausted psychological explanations of healing as insufficient or inadequate to define the construct despite years of training, teaching, and practicing with access to that discipline (Dossey 2001; Frattaroli 2001; Herman 1992; Jung 2006 [1957]; Maslow 1999; Whitfield 1987). As an anthropologist, I observed the social practices and interactions that shape healing relationships, relationships that connect the individual to our cultural world. Social practices can be observed and therefore have a greater scientific claim to define a construct in the real world.

The ethnographer as data collection instrument

"When it's done right, participant observation turns field workers into instruments of data collection and data analysis" (Bernard 2002: 324). This statement implies participant observation can be done incorrectly and result in inaccurate data. The validity of this research depends on my qualifications to do participant observation. Raymond Madden voices a common methodological concern: reflexivity, or the ability to prevent writing oneself into the data unknowingly (Madden 2013 [2010]: 2). Prior to any formal anthropological training, I came equipped with "reflexivity," a necessary skill for ethnographers. I spent six years becoming a certified Balint leader, a group process based on psychoanalytic principles; two of those years were spent with individual supervision (American Balint Society). During that time, I practiced the cognitive skills to monitor two, three, or four things simultaneously in real time. A Balint leader must observe the speech, symbolic attributes of speech, body language or proxemics, emotions, shared emotions, and group dynamics, all for discerning the "story" of the case as the group participants re-enact it. Psychoanalytic frameworks have the added benefit of leaving no doubt about distinguishing self from other. That is definitional of transference and countertransference. Distinguishing self from other is required to do anthropological work. Ethnographers must also monitor multiple social spaces and levels of analysis simultaneously. Figure 1.1 is a metaphor for the reflexivity required.

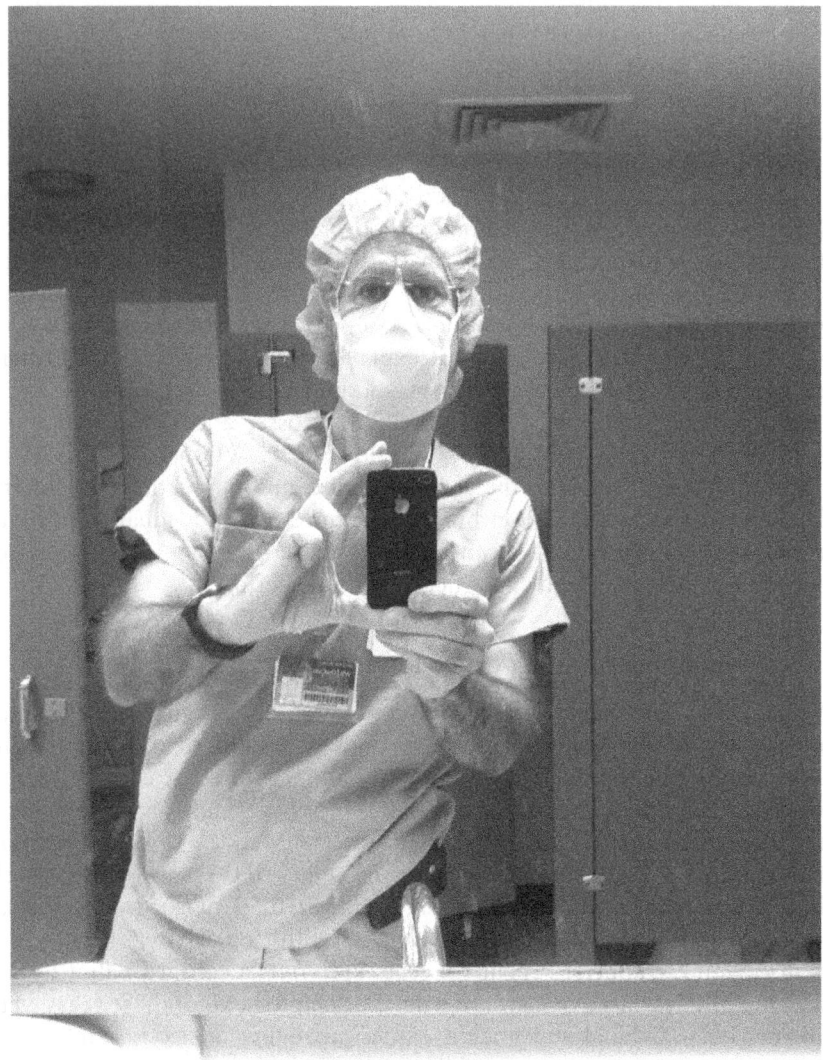

Figure 1.1 Self-portrait of ethnographer

Figure 1.1 demonstrates the distance from my retina to my hand, the distance from the camera to the mirror as recorded on the screen of the camera, the distance from my retina to the image on the camera screen, and the distance from my retina to the mirror – all these observations occurred simultaneously. Ethnography requires awareness of multiple perspectives simultaneously.

Early in my anthropological training, a mentor handed me a journal article co-authored by Arthur Kleinman (Smilkstein et al. 1981). The implication was that my biomedical training prevented me from becoming a legitimate anthropologist or social scientist. Although I said nothing at the time, I had read that article contemporaneously upon publication and the biopsychosocial model was part of my training from my youth (Engel 1977; Engel 1996). I have spent thirty years listening, pondering the meaning, and struggling to understand patients and their stories. Yet, respected anthropologists told me I would never be able to see cultural information because "You think like a doctor." In fact, this fascination with the duality of being both an anthropologist and a master clinician has been a matter of persistent curiosity since the day I first met an anthropologist; the fascination continues until today. I was always in the marked category. Professors would stop mid-sentence and say, "Oh, you're *that* student." Other anthropologists used my medical background as a challenge to the validity of my anthropological work because of my assumed bias toward defending biomedicine. Nancy Chen describes similar complexities of being a Chinese American working as an ethnographer in China (Chen 2003: 5). Long ago, I decided this was much more of a reflection of the culture of academia than anything to do with my work or me. Actually, my pragmatic realism allows me to accept simultaneously both biomedical and sociocultural perspectives about reality. I understand science is a cultural production (Canguilhem 1991 [1978]; Latour 1999; Lewontin 1992 [1991]).

Perhaps I can best illustrate with an example that predates this research. "Grand Rounds" is a medical education tradition (one might say ritual), where an intern, the least senior doctor, presents to the entire department a difficult case seen on the hospital wards that week. There ensues an exhaustive discussion of the every possible diagnosis and the audience challenges the presenter with questions of all sorts. Why were certain tests ordered or not ordered, physical exam findings, and book knowledge of rare diseases are all part of the enactment. The intern usually spends enormous time and effort preparing for this spectacle because the chair of the department attends, as well as most of the senior faculty who did not even participate in caring for the patient. Of course no matter how prepared, the process "teaches" by pointing out mistakes (Brancati 1989). The stated goal is to "prove" the correct diagnosis.

I was present for many such conferences. As a doctor, I typically could discern the actual diagnosis within five to ten minutes by juggling the positive and negative space of the diagnosis as a cognitive construct (Edwards 1979). The remaining fifty minutes rely on a system of diagnosis referred to in the medical community as an "exhaustive" diagnostic approach; I was typically bored throughout that part – again, a symptom of my pragmatism. As an anthropologist, I watched who was allowed to speak and when, the cultural capital of superior medical knowledge and how that "knowledge" determined the "reality" of facts, the delicate balance of demonstrating competence while fearing humiliation in a social setting, administrative and cultural power structures and how they interacted within the case discussion. I witnessed what Pierre Bourdieu and Jean-Claude Passeron called *Reproduction in Education, Society and Culture* (Bourdieu and Passeron 1990 [1970]). On one notable occasion, my diagnosis differed from a powerful faculty physician who had originally trained as a surgeon. As such, his knowledge of anatomy was unquestioned. He deployed that knowledge by reviewing x-rays to support his diagnosis. Although the entire department agreed with his diagnosis, after the conference I walked down the hall to the radiology department and they confirmed that my interpretation was correct; this meant twenty-five other people had a different impression of that diagnostic "reality" based on cultural practices. During such episodes, I am fully a clinician and fully an anthropologist.

The methodologically important part of that example is that I am aware of when I "cognitively code-switch" from doctor to anthropologist. I approached this research purely as an anthropologist. I rarely comment on something from a doctor's perspective, but I always declare when I do that. This is ethnography.

Just as anthropologists have questioned my veracity because of medical training, doctors question my veracity if I try to explain the sociocultural aspects of behaviors in a clinical setting. Mary Douglas would call me dirt. Oh well. My eclectic lifelong learning agenda has exposed me to many disciplines other than medicine and anthropology. I love statistics. Others comment that I am odd, but I can "see" statistical distributions in social settings; I can estimate the probability of events in my head and recognize when social behaviors are not randomly distributed. I have studied health law, accounting, human resource management, psychology, economics, psychometrics, art history, evidence-based medicine, and other intellectual pursuits. None of these disciplines has a unique window on reality. Although the jargon varies, many constructs have a common core underlying how people understand the world.

Ethnographer as social actor

Throughout the course of fieldwork, I was vigilant to monitor my position as a social actor. I knew I needed to guard against informants perceiving me as having medical knowledge. An anthropologist must start with the assumption that they know nothing and ask those in the culture under study to teach them. It is more difficult to function as an anthropologist in "one's own culture." It is much easier to compare the *other* to the culture of origin while studying an unfamiliar culture.

I was quite successful at being perceived as "uninformed" by always taking the "power down" position when gathering data. My informants treated me as a medical student, a family medicine physician learning urology, a PhD student, an interloper or voyeur, a pet, an uninitiated observer, or the object of teasing. I was usually ignored, remediated, teased, taught, or given gifts of insight. Unexpectedly, I encountered occasional fear about collecting "evaluative" data, which hospital administrators could misuse. I was diligent about reinforcing the non-evaluative nature of anthropology as a social science. Those in the field rarely excluded me from participation; the only two occasions I recall were a VIP patient and a matter of litigation. I helped in the daily tasks consistent with my "novice level" of experience. On one occasion, I drove around town to retrieve a cell phone for one of the faculty physicians so that the clinic could stay on schedule.

I am thankful for the participants allowing me access and establishing rapport sufficient to acquire the data. I quite easily reached that ethnographic "sweet spot" where I was present, but ignored as part of the surroundings – like a piece of furniture. One of the faculty physicians had seen me hanging around at various locations for over a year. We were talking in the hallway. I was thanking him for his participation, and he pointed and touched my photo identification badge with the corporate logo that clearly labeled me as an MD. He asked me if that was a joke. I said, "No, I'm a family medicine physician."

He was taken aback and then said, "I'm sorry," and went on to apologize for I don't know what, but I imagined for not treating me as a physician in front of the patients. It was obvious that he was oblivious to the fact that I was a doctor for the previous year. He was apologetic, but I was pleased that my social role or presumed knowledge had not tainted data collection during participant observation. He then continued to joke and tease me, saying, "Between me and the nurse, we have a sociology degree and a psychology degree, so you can't fool us – we're a tough crowd."

When in social areas not directly related to patient care, the medical assistants were extremely friendly and we all engaged in chitchat. At certain intervals, I would provide lunch simply to socialize. This allowed for data collection in a very informal manner because we were essentially breaking bread together. When I was with the resident physicians, they treated me at about the level of the medical student in terms of hierarchy. There were many times the residents were not directly supervised by someone higher in the hierarchy, and at those times, I felt a strong degree of affinity toward them, a sense of belonging. This also extended to the urology outpatient office. When I was absent more than a couple of weeks, I would miss being there and would make a point to stop by simply to say hello. These episodes occurred when I was in the other field site locations. In the presence of attending physicians, I was treated like they treated the residents, tolerated and guided as a learner. Throughout the entire data collection, I maintained contact with that initial site.

Validity

During my anthropological training, I attended sessions where parsed transcripts were pile-sorted into "themes" by three different anthropologists simultaneously. Qualitative researchers use triangulation as a proxy for validity in qualitative research. Although I can accept the methodological process has some utility, I always questioned the validity of the method. When I discuss theory of the mind in the next chapter, it will become clear that this method of "triangulating data" could also be seen as a cultural practice of groupthink,[2] relegating the findings to an emic-only perspective.

External validity

I believe a far superior method of triangulating ethnographic data is to triangulate between the individual body, the cultural body, and the body politic (Scheper-Hughes and Lock 1987). The two ethnographies I'm aware of that accomplished this task the best are the works by Nancy Scheper-Hughes (Scheper-Hughes 1992) and Fay Ginsburg (Ginsburg 1989). More typically, ethnographies thoroughly cover two of the three and hint at the third. Two examples that emphasize the individual body and cultural body include those by Carol Stack (1974) and Howard Becker et al. (1961). Examples of ethnographies that emphasize the body politic and the cultural body include those by Matthew Kohrman (2005) and Adriana Petryna (2002). I mention these ethnographies for illustrative purposes only. The ideal is to describe all three "bodies" comprehensively, but in practice, most ethnography accomplishes two of the three. My research question related to cultural practices that happened in the clinical exam room, so my descriptions emphasize the individual body and the cultural body. As I said, this data was purely anthropological based on the paradigm of exploring, discovering, understanding, and describing. For validity, I felt it important to "triangulate" this data with components of the body politic. My original ethnographic data on the body politic was collected during the project and I use it to provide sociopolitical context. The value to this project is to realize that these societal-level concerns are indeed present in the everyday and mundane practice of medicine, triangulating the ethnographic data for establishing validity. In Appendix A, I record personal narratives which demonstrate how individuals have incorporated the cultural information into their personal stories. Appendix B was collected six to nine months after the fieldwork and I was shocked at how well doctors discussing their work corroborated my participant observation data.

Internal validity

I had been in the field for a year, and began sharing the initial findings with the funding agency, members in my field site, colleagues, friends, and described details about how Michel Foucault's "clinical gaze" is a three-dimensional cognition reconstructed from two-dimensional CT[3] and MRI[4] scan images. I explained this all as if it was a profound discovery. For me it was an extremely exciting finding as an anthropologist. It was not until almost the conclusion of my fieldwork and at least six to nine months after I had sufficient data to begin sharing this concept with others that I had an *Aha!* moment and realized that what I had "discovered" in my fieldwork was something that I myself have done hundreds of times in clinical practice. The sequence of these two "discoveries" matters. If I had said to myself, "I do this when I practice medicine; let me see if I can find it in this other clinical setting," then the criticism that I could only find biased data because I was a physician-ethnographer would be true. The fact that I "discovered" this practice after closely observing it hundreds of times in the field while being unaware of the same cognitive processes in my own clinical work is merely a reflection that we are all unaware of our own culture (Peacock 1986: 4).

Reliability

Internal reliability

Ethnography is not known for reliability – the ability to measure something twice and get the same answer both times. I did, however have experiences that led me to believe there is reliability to my major findings. In the course of fieldwork, I wrote a massive amount of field notes. I had finished fieldwork, analysis, and writing, and it was time to clean up. I came across old field notes from very early in my fieldwork that I overlooked (and were therefore not included in my analysis and report). When I re-read them, I realized that I had written and described in great detail the same social practices that later became part of the analysis and report. But contemporaneously while writing the field notes I never recognized the social practice. A psychometrician would call this a "hold out sample" and report it as a marker of reliability.

External reliability

During the 2016 Olympics in Rio de Janeiro, I was watching television and saw many sports medicine advertisements. Again, I observed CT and MRI images deployed in the same way I describe with my ethnographic data. I saw doctors "flipping through" two-dimensional images in rapid sequence – but let me save the description of that practice for later. Suffice it to say, I describe in my data the same cultural practices advertising agencies replicate to sell medical services. Seeing the same cultural practices in different places and different times is a marker for reliability.

Generalizability

Ethnographic data is known for its granular detail; the data itself is typically not generalizable. The theoretical insights generated are the generalizable portion of ethnography. Incorporating new theoretical insights with the existing anthropological canon is a stronger form of generalizability.

Because my field site was a surgical subspecialty, others have questioned the relevance to medical subspecialties. I appeal to Michel Foucault's *Birth of the Clinic* (Foucault 1973, 1994).

He described the origins of Western medicine arising from cadaver dissection illuminating modern human anatomy and the origin of the "laboratory" in the clinic. I believe both are present in medicine and surgical subspecialties; it is merely a matter of emphasis. Both anatomy and the "laboratory" are present in my data, as I describe urology (a surgical subspecialty) and oncology (a medical subspecialty). I chose to organize the text with anatomy, but clearly the "laboratory" can be found throughout both disciplines. Using Foucault's description and my data, I would call anatomy and physiology the "king and queen of the medical sciences." My license to practice medicine is a cultural artifact that declares I am a "physician and surgeon."

Fieldwork

Field site selection

I chose the fieldwork site based on the study design. The attributes of the setting itself contributed to the observation of data. The discipline of urology has tremendous conflict, diversity of opinion, passionate debate, and a standard of care that is fluctuating. The current practice of urology is not a stable social system, and the areas of disagreement highlight and bring forth key cultural facts in a readily accessible manner. I am referring to the controversy regarding PSA[5] as well as radical robotic prostatectomy and so forth; thus, I expected to observe rich discursive work, a good sampling frame based on my research question.

Another attribute of the fieldwork site was that it involved a post-graduate medical training program and in that way was an example of rapid cycle cultural replication. The first-year resident (post-graduate, year two) enters as the neophyte and through the course of the program emerges as an independent practitioner. From the participant observer's point of view, "training" is a process of socialization into the cultural norms of the practice of urology. The rapid replication of culture in a setting of conflicting standards of practice amplifies the ability to observe cultural facts in the field setting.

Informed consent

The institutional review board approved this project. Every patient received an information sheet, as did participants in social settings. Once an operating room nurse who read the information sheet asked, "Who are you? What is this?" I was with a group of resident physicians who quickly came to my rescue, at which point she said, "If you're with them, that's good enough for me." I obtained written consent for audio-recorded ethnographic interviews.

Data collection

The vast majority of my data came from participant observation. Because I was observing clinical encounters, it was vital that I not disrupt the actual work of the doctor or interfere with the encounter from the patient's perspective. For making scratch notes, I used Moleskine notebooks that were 3.5 × 5.5 inches with sixty-four plain pages per notebook. The size allowed me to hide it comfortably in the palm of my hand while observing, as well as to store the notebook in almost any pocket. This was more optimal than obvious data collection tools (such as an iPad) that would stick out as foreign to the field setting.

For every observation session, I dictated the scratch notes immediately after the observation, most often in the parking lot nearest to the field site; this provided privacy and freedom from interruption and allowed me to capture the experience close to the real-time occurrence. Dictating immediately after observation also allowed short-term memory to augment the scratch notes while contextualizing the observations. I used an Olympus Digital voice recorder (DM-420) for dictating. I was careful to dictate field notes that were observational in nature with as much detail as possible. I used Dragon NaturallySpeaking 11 to transcribe these notes.

Occasionally, I observed something that I as the ethnographer had an opinion about the meaning of an event. I was diligent to segregate my opinions in the notes with the heading "observer's reflection" so that the actual observations were not conflated with my internal thoughts that occurred during the period of observation. On occasions when I had an emotional reaction during observation, that was also recorded in the segregated notation portion of the field notes.

I conducted ethnographic interviews with patients concurrent with the participant observation and I detail some of them in Appendix A. Interviews with administrators produced little of value. I interviewed knowledgeable physicians familiar with the societal issues during fieldwork. However, I conducted the three ethnographic interviews with Dr. Jeffries, Dr. Stein, and Dr. Spangler (three principal key informants during participant observation) after conclusion of the participant observation. I chose this design purposely to verify and confirm that the data from participant observation was correct and that I had not missed important aspects of the cultural practices I had observed.

Recording conversational data

Because I was trying to identify the discursive maneuvers in a clinical encounter, my scratch notes recorded the speaker sequence, the word choice, and the conversational content by rapidly recording turn-taking with opening quotation marks and skipping to the next line when a new speaker started or indicating the speaker with one initial of their code name. I concurrently abbreviated sentence structure and content in shorthand. As mentioned, I dictated these conversations into my field notes almost immediately while I still had an intact short-term memory of the conversation, allowing me to include almost all of the conversational details. I occasionally missed a portion of a conversation, but incomplete notations were not included in the results. In this way, I was able to reconstruct large segments of conversation without being overly intrusive and using an audio recording device. Because the observational data is dialogue of natural speech by the participants, it contains a fair amount of medical jargon. I provide endnotes in the manuscript to translate "medicalese" into discipline-specific English. For readers who might be doctors, I also use the endnotes to clarify anthropological jargon. Because language reflects cultural categories, I needed to mentally code-switch as I looked for the data that would answer my research question.

Creating mental memos

As part of collecting field notes, there was the concurrent experience of reflection and pondering both what I observed and what the meaning of what I observed was. Typically, I would take a two-mile walk, lasting about ninety minutes, and simply let my thoughts flow over the experiences of fieldwork. The *Aha!* moment I described occurred during this reflective time. This dedicated reflection time occurred in equal measure to the time I actually spent at the field sites. It was during these times that I would formulate the ongoing ethnographic hypotheses that I would then go back and confirm or deny with further observations.

The fieldwork site and the metaphor of "the village"

I used the metaphor of "the village" to trace the social spaces of the key participants. I observed the key informants "at home" and also everywhere they traveled throughout the "village." This meant I explored several different hospitals, outpatient clinics, and met everyone with whom they interacted. I was fortunate that the index site (Maplewood Clinic, an outpatient urology office) incorporated the workplace of both the "chief" and the "medicine man"; namely, the chairperson of the department of urology and the residency program director both used the index site as part of their clinical practice.

The methodological purpose of spending enough time at the index site was to form hypotheses so that subsequently, when I went to other portions of "the village," I could try to confirm observations made earlier. This confirmation of the same ethnographic data in a different location with other people was a form of validity for this study. I was able to confirm the observations in every other site of "the village." The process of taking field notes described earlier included enough detail that I was able to not only confirm observations going forward in time, but I was also able to look back at earlier field notes and confirm observations retrospectively that were not appreciated at the time of data collection. Again, the process of understanding the cultural information was cumulative, and I confirmed observations in both an antegrade fashion and a retrograde fashion, a marker of validity.

After starting at the index site, I sequentially added these new sites while maintaining contact with the index site and concluding by completing some of the final observations at the index site itself. It was a complete urological experience from multiple different perspectives. At each site, I had to ask permission and gain access. In terms of "exploring the village," I reached saturation having visited every place on multiple occasions.

Visits to the fieldwork site occurred approximately twice weekly, every week, or every other week. There was never an extended gap or lack of contact with the fieldwork site. If I was away for an extended period of time, I would stop in and say hello, just to let the people I was working with know that I was still thinking about them. Likewise, if I changed locations, I notified participants where I was and when I would return. The amount of time spent at a site was typically four hours or one-half of a workday, the typical length of an outpatient clinic session. Other observations were from twelve to fourteen hours, particularly when the fieldwork site was in the hospital.

Gaining access to the field site

I had chosen a urological training program for methodological reasons. I showed up at the tertiary care hospital and asked how to find that office only to be told there was none on site. It turned out that the urology residency program merely used that hospital as a training location. I next went to the university clinic and was chased away by the nurse administrator who was protective of space and clinic operations related to patient flow. Eventually I found an administrative office and made an appointment with Dr. Jeffries. He wrote the letter of introduction to his colleagues. Dr. Stein did refer to the letter once about a year and a half later, saying, "That's the only reason I allowed you to observe my clinic." Asking permission took about six months prior to what I refer to as "entrance to the field." Dr. Jeffries invited me to his clinic where he saw patients and this was my foot in the door, as I quickly met everybody in the fieldwork site. Eventually I collected observations in all locations, including the site the nurse administrator initially denied access. I had to fill out bureaucratic forms and obtain permissions from multiple institutions. I had three "employee photo name badges" and had four tests for tuberculosis in one year (typically, doctors are only required to do this once yearly). I do not include any of these experiences as data, because the research question was focused on the doctor-patient interactions.

Analysis

The field notes and interviews resulted in a large body of textual data. Each fieldwork experience resulted in a primary document that was included in a single hermeneutic unit in ATLAS.ti v6.2. The codes themselves came from the theoretical frame, which I also wrote prior to entering the field. I used a couple of codes from prior ethnographic fieldwork I had done in teaching hospitals (Meza and Rohn 2007). I did not use any "emergent codes" for analysis because I wanted the theoretical frame to drive the analysis (Appendix C).

I wrote the definition of the codes used for qualitative analysis prior to coding any of the data. Initial review of the data started with generating reports of individual codes to understand the range of content in the data set. I then generated crosstabs queries of paired codes. I parsed the crosstab queries and used pile sorting to generate initial themes. I proceeded to look at interactions between the themes and looked for a "bigger picture" from an analytic perspective. While working with these themes, I recognized the pattern "ritual" that I had not previously appreciated. I then re-read much of what was written on narrative healing, including Kleinman's *Illness Narratives* and Mattingly's *Healing Dramas and Clinical Plots: The Narrative Structure of Experience*. I found these two texts to be most compelling. I probably read and re-read each a dozen times during the analysis. Sometimes I perseverated on a single sentence. Unrecognized by me prior to that point, they both recognized the clinical encounter as ritual. However, neither anthropologist expanded on narrative as ritual. This led to my re-examination of the foundational literature on healing rituals (Fortes 1987; Pritchard 1976; Rivers 2001 [1924]; Turner 1969).

I re-examined my original theoretical grounding for this research project. I wanted to understand the clinical encounter in the way Mattingly described: "the narrative structure of action and experience" (1998: 2). Most anthropological literature on healing rituals has a dominant symbolic interpretation. I merged the theoretical concepts of narrative, theory of the mind, and ritual as an adaptation of Mattingly's work and argue that the clinical encounter is the narrative structure of ritual experience. This has the parsimony of argument that joint attention (to the ritual experience) is a narrative cultural production that I believe both Mattingly and Tomasello could endorse. I found support for the foundational descriptions of the healing ritual in the works of others (Dow 1986; Frank and Frank 1991; Milne and Howard 2000; Moerman 1979).

In Chapter 2, I report my original theoretical frame. Beginning in Chapter 3, I present ethnographic data. To simulate the process of analysis, I present a discussion of ritual as it relates to my initial theoretical frame as an interval discussion of theory in the midst of the ethnographic data (Chapter 9) and use this heuristic to present more of the ethnographic data. The organization of the book reflects the analytic journey of the project.

Both anthropology and family medicine self-define as "generalists," meaning part of their task is to integrate disparate and large data sets. Within this ethnography, I started by merging narrative theory with concepts from cognitive anthropology to achieve a parsimonious theoretical frame to do the research. During the analysis, I once again merged anthropological understandings of ritual to my original theoretical frame. I find evidence for this in the works of Mattingly and Kleinman, but push this theoretical exploration further. I hope I have adequately supported these theoretical claims with ethnographic data. I find these concepts fit together nicely and helped me understand the social practices between doctors and patients within my own epistemological perspective. More importantly, I satisfied myself that I answered the research question that had engaged me throughout many years.

Notes

1

> *Pragmatic Realism*: The doctrine that knowledge comes by way of action, that to know is to act by hypotheses which result in successful adaption or resolve practical difficulties. According to pragmatic realism, the mind is not outside the realm of nature; in experience the organism and the world are at one; the theories of knowledge which follow the alleged dualism between the objective and subjective worlds are false. Ideas and knowledge are instruments for activity and not spectators of an outside realm. — V. F.
> Dagobert D. Runes, *Dictionary of Philosophy*, 1942.
> www.ditext.com/runes/p.html (accessed January 20, 2017)

2 "The practice of approaching problems or issues as matters that are best dealt with by consensus of a group rather than by individuals acting independently; conformity." www.dictionary.com/browse/groupthink?s=t (accessed January 20, 2017).
3 An acronym for computed tomography. A tomogram is a slice, in this case, a slice of the body as reconstituted with a computer using x-ray data.
4 An acronym for magnetic resonance imaging. This uses the electrical valence of electrons in the body and disrupts them with an extremely powerful magnet. When the magnet is disengaged, the electrons snap back into place and generate small amounts of radiation that "resonates" and therefore measureable. This also generates a tomographic image, generally of higher quality than the CT.
5 An acronym for prostatic specific antigen, a blood test purportedly used to screen for prostate cancer.

References

The American-Balint-Society. http://americanbalintsociety.org/, accessed April 9, 2018.

Becker, Howard S., et al. 1961. *Boys in White: Student Culture in Medical School*. New Brunswick, NJ: Transaction.

Bernard, H. Russel. 2002. *Research Methods in Anthropology, Qualitative and Quantitative Approaches*. Walnut Creek, CA: AltaMira Press.

Bourdieu, Pierre, and Jean-Claude Passeron. 1990 [1970]. *Reproduction in Education, Society and Culture*. R. Nice, transl. London: Sage.

Brancati, Frederick L. 1989. The Art of Pimping. *JAMA* 262(1):89–90.

Cahoone, Lawrence. 2010. *The Modern Intellectual Tradition: From Descartes to Derrida*. Chantilly, VA: Great Courses.

Canguilhem, Georges. 1991 [1978]. *The Normal and the Pathological*. New York: Zone Books.

Chen, Nancy N. 2003. *Breathing Spaces: Qigong, Psychiatry, and Healing in China*. New York: Columbia University Press.

Cohen, Deborah J., and Benjamin F. Crabtree. 2008. Evaluative Criteria for Qualitative Research in Health Care: Controversies and Recommendations. *Annals of Family Medicine* 6:331–339.

Dossey, Larry. 2001. *Healing Beyond the Body: Medicine and the Infinite Reach of the Mind*. Boston: Shambhala.

Dow, James. 1986. Universal Aspects of Symbolic Healing: A Theoretical Synthesis. American Anthropologist. *New Series* 88(1):56–69.

Edwards, Betty. 1979. *Drawing on the Right Side of the Brain: A Course in Enhancing Creativity and Artistic Confidence*. Los Angeles: J.P. Tarcher.

Engel, George. 1977. The Need for a New Medical Model: A Challenge for Biomedicine. *Science* 196:129–136.

———. 1996. From Biomedical to Biopsychosocial: Being Scientific in the Human Domain. Families. *Systems & Health* 14(4):425–433.

Ewing, Katherine P. 1990. The Illusion of Wholeness: Culture, Self, and the Experience of Inconsistency. *Ethos* 18(3):251–278.

Fortes, Meyer. 1987. *Religion, Morality, and the Person: Essays on Tallensi Religion*. Cambridge: Cambridge University Press.

Foucault, Michel. 1973[1994]. *The Birth of the Clinic: An Archeology of Medical Perception*. New York: Vintage Books.

Frank, Jerome D., and Julia B. Frank. 1991. *Persuasion & Healing: A Comparative Study of Psychotherapy*. Baltimore: Johns Hopkins University Press.

Frattaroli, Elio. 2001. *Healing the Soul in the Age of the Brain*. New York: Viking.

Ginsburg, Faye D. 1989. *Contested Lives: The Abortion Debate in an American Community*. Berkeley: University of California Press.

Goldman, Steven L. 2006. *Science Wars: What Scientists Know and How They Know It*. Chantilly, VA: Great Courses.

Herman, Judith Lewis. 1992. *Trauma and Recovery*. New York: Basic Books.

Jung, Carl G. 2006 [1957]. *The Undiscovered Self*. New York: New American Library.

Kasser, Jeffrey L. 2006. *The Philosophy of Science*. Chantilly, VA: Great Courses.

Kohrman, Matthew. 2005. *Bodies of Difference: Experiences of Disability and Institutional Advocacy in the Making of Modern China*. Berkeley: University of California Press.

Latour, Bruno. 1999. *Pandora's Hope*. Cambridge: Harvard University Press.

Lewontin, Richard C. 1992 [1991]. *Biology as Ideology: The Doctrine of DNA*. New York: HarperCollins.

Madden, Raymond. 2013 [2010]. *Being Ethnographic: A Guide to the Theory and Practice of Ethnography*. London: SAGE.

Maslow, Abraham H. 1999. *Toward a Psychology of Being*. New York: John Wiley & Sons.

Mattingly, Cheryl. 1998. *Healing Dramas and Clinical Plots: The Narrative Structure of Experience*. Cambridge: Cambridge University Press.

Mattingly, Cheryl, and Linda C. Garro, eds. 2000. *Narrative and the Cultural Construction of Illness and Healing*. Berkeley: University of California Press.

Meza, James, and Edward Rohn. 2007. Power and Professionalism in Medical Education. *In Rethinking Health, Culture, and Society. Physician-Scholars in the Social Sciences and Medical Humanities*. Chicago.

Milne, Derek, and Wilson Howard. 2000. Rethinking the Role of Diagnosis in Navajo Religious Healing. *Medical Anthropology Quarterly* 14(4):543–570.

Moerman, Daniel. 1979. Anthropology of Symbolic Healing. *Current Anthropology* 20(1).

Murphy, Yolanda, and Robert F. Murphy. 2004. *Women of the Forest*. New York: Columbia University Press.

Peacock, James. 1986. *The Anthropological Lens: Harsh Light, Soft Focus*. Cambridge: Cambridge University Press.

Petryna, Adriana. 2002. *Life Exposed: Biological Citizens After Chernobyl*. Princeton, NJ: Princeton University Press.

Pritchard, E., and E. Evans. 1976. *Witchcraft, Oracles, and Magic Among the Azande*. Oxford: Clarendon Press.

Rivers, W.H.R. 2001 [1924]. *Medicine, Magic, and Religion*. London: Routledge Classics.

Robinson, Daniel N. 2004. *The Great Ideas of Philosophy*. Chantilly, VA: Great Courses.

Rudnytsky, Peter, and Rita Charon, eds. 2008. *Psychoanalysis and Narrative Medicine*. Albany: State University of New York Press.

Scheper-Hughes, Nancy. 1992. *Death Without Weeping: The Violence of Everyday Life in Brazil*. Berkeley: University of California Press.

Scheper-Hughes, Nancy, and M.M. Lock. 1987. The Mindful Body: A Prolegomenon to Future Work in Medical Anthropology. *Medical Anthropology Quarterly* 1:6–41.

Smilkstein, Gabriel, et al. 1981. The Clinical Social Science Conference in Biopsychosocial Teaching. *Journal of Family Practice* 12(2):347–353.

Stack, Carol. 1974. *All Our Kin*. New York: Basic Books.

Turner, Victor. 1969. *The Ritual Process*. Chicago: Aldine.

Whitfield, Charles L. 1987. *Healing the Child Within: Discovery and Recovery for Adult Children of Dysfunctional Families*. Deerfield Beach, FL: Health Communications.

2 The theoretical frame

Theory helps organize the analysis of the ethnographic data; I selected narrative theorists that support the epistemology of pragmatic realism. My epistemological perspective has foundational implications for this study. Who is the narrator? Is the story true; is the story a form of reality? Is anthropology a science or a relativistic story about others? Most narrative texts acknowledge the ambiguity by using words such as "body-self," "self-story," or "body-self-story." Indeed, it is hard to find an anthropological text on healing that does not include the word "self." These hyphenated constructs beg the question of what or who is healed? What is healing? Claims that the doctor is the socially designated "healer" have face validity (Frank and Frank 1991). Yet, contemporary ethnographic narrative healing studies rarely include the doctor and the social practices in which the doctor participates. This book hopes to begin to fill that gap. I present ethnographic data within an anthropological framework. I intend to honor the traditions of the discipline even though I present a very different perspective of narrative healing. After changing the perspective on narrative studies of healing, I will retrace prior works and try to demonstrate how this work and those prior contributors can be viewed as a synthetic whole – indeed, that explanatory power is part of the pragmatism I espouse. Although a thorough analysis of the self could take many volumes, I provide a narrow definition of self that includes consciousness and free will based on recognized foundational thinkers in narrative theory. Other prominent anthropologists explore the outer edges of these questions (Murphey and Throop 2010). My theoretical conceptualization and epistemology are critical to the analysis, interpretation, and concluding thoughts in this ethnography.

It is important to understand that I confine my argument to the cultural context of Western (cosmopolitan) medicine. Anthropologists honor the belief systems of other cultures and I make no claims to generalize these arguments to cross-cultural studies on healing. My pragmatism demands anthropological answers that enable me to become a better doctor.

Theory of the mind – differentiating person from self

In *The Cultural Origins of Human Cognition*, Michael Tomasello (1999) summarizes his arguments based on his prior investigations. He claims the cognitive phenomena he describes form the basis for all future cultural development in human beings. Specifically, Tomasello reviews three types of learning: imitative learning, instructed learning, and collaborative learning. He then states:

> These three types of cultural learning are made possible by a single very special form of social cognition, namely, the ability of the individual organisms to understand conspecifics as beings like themselves who have intentional and mental life like their own.
>
> (Tomasello 1999: 5)

His argument proceeds that natural selection is unable to explain the rapid cultural developments of *Homo sapiens* because there is simply not enough time for the myriad of evolutionary changes to take place. Based on this simple cognitive argument, he describes the ratchet effect:

> The process of cumulative cultural evolution requires not only creative invention but also, and just as importantly, faithful social transmission that can work as a ratchet to prevent slippage backward – so that the newly invented artifact or practice preserves its new and improved form at least somewhat faithfully until a further modification or improvement comes along.
>
> (Tomasello 1999: 5)

He goes on to state:

> Multiple individuals create something together that no one individual could have created on its own. These special powers come directly from the fact that as one human being is learning "through" another, she identifies with that person and his intentional and sometimes mental states.
>
> (Tomasello 1999: 6)

Tomasello's argument is that cultural development and the genesis of culture itself is based on the premise described, broadly acknowledged in other disciplines as "the theory of the mind." Tomasello describes individual human growth and development in the mental cognitive domain, stating:

> The child comes to experience herself as an intentional agent – that is, a being whose behavioral and attentional strategies are organized by goals – and so she automatically sees other beings with whom she identifies in the same terms. Later in ontogeny, the child comes to experience herself as a mental agent – that is a being with thoughts and beliefs that may differ from those of other people as well as from reality – and so from that time on she will seek conspecifics in these new terms.
>
> (Tomasello 1999: 14–15)

Tomasello describes accumulated human history as "processes of cultural learning and internalization by which developing individuals learn to use and then internalized aspects of the collaborative products created by conspecifics" (Tomasello 1999: 15). Tomasello describes an anthropological self as mental agent with thoughts and beliefs, derived from conspecifics, but are nonetheless unique, evidenced by the fact that the individual mental agent evaluates self from other with an understanding of the other. *When I use the term self, I refer to this definition.* I stipulate this definition for the sake of developing an argument about healing, well aware that others may have differing opinions. Embedded within the definition is a relationship between the self and society, a key argument for defining healing.

Tomasello later recapitulates:

> This is the uniqueness from which all else flows, as it enables infants to exploit a novel source of information about other persons: the analogy to the self. At around nine months of age, analogizing self and other persons enables infants to attribute to other persons the same kinds of intentionality in which they themselves are just beginning to engage (and they may also analogize to the self, somewhat inappropriately, in their causal reasoning about why inanimate objects behave as they do).
>
> (Tomasello 1999: 213)

This goal-oriented and causal reasoning allows for the development of shared narrative – in the context of this research, a shared diagnosis narrative. It also allows for a shared narrative conveying intentionality, a necessary precursor of transformative powers.

The second major concept outlined by Tomasello is the emergence of joint attention. By careful and detailed exposition, Tomasello describes normal human development, beginning at approximately 9 to 12 months of age. At that age,

> a new set of behaviors emerge that are not dyadic, . . . but are triadic in the sense that they involve the coordination of their interaction with objects and people, resulting in a referential triangle of child, adult, and the object or event to which they share attention.
>
> (Tomasello 1999: 62)

Tomasello describes this joint attention as a uniquely human communicative behavior. While joint attention is required for cultural learning, I will examine a very narrow focus of cultural learning described as communicating the diagnosis narrative by joint attention to a specific object: the three-dimensional computer image of a diseased organ. Narratives are stories; stories are cultural communication from one human to others. Thus, doctors share a diagnosis narrative – primarily with the patient, but also with the entire community participating in medical-surgical therapy. For now, it is important to understand that basic human cognitions described by Tomasello are essential to clinical encounters. Expanding the argument, Tomasello elaborates:

> Narratives add more complexity still, as they string together simple events in ways that invite causal and intentional analysis, and indeed explicitly symbolized causal and intentional marking, to make them coherent. And extended discourse and other kinds of social interactions with adults lead children into even more esoteric cognitive spaces, as they enable them to understand conflicting perspectives on things that must be reconciled in some way.
>
> (Tomasello 1999: 214)

This research study depends on the ability of the doctor to construct a diagnosis narrative and convey that cognition to the patient, to persuade the patient to accept the diagnosis narrative despite potential conflicting explanations, and subsequently to act on the diagnosis with a therapeutic maneuver. This shared activity demonstrates "learning through the other" and creates a shared narrative between the doctor and the patient.

Theoretically, I find anthropological theory of narrative based on these cognitive foundations. Throughout the literature, the contested role of self as it relates to culture cannot stray too far from those attributes of humans that make culture possible. Starting with joint attention between two humans and expanding that concept through shared understandings by many people, these social narratives are a form of pragmatic realism – the culture at large accepts preferred narratives only if they have pragmatic value.

Personal experience and narrative

William Labov's sociolinguistic observations of natural speech provide one of the basic definitions of narrative. His work is highly consonant with the findings of Tomasello. He states, "[Human] communication may draw upon the fundamental capacity to transfer experience from one person to another through oral narratives of personal experience" (Labov 2010: 546). This is one-half of the ratchet effect referred to by Tomasello. In the preceding quote, it is important to note that narrative, as defined by Labov, is preceded by experience and subsequently "told" to a conspecific. His contribution is to elaborate the fundamental structure of narrative (as opposed to the cognitive attributes allowing narrative). Labov states, "Narrative structure is established by the existence of a temporal juncture between two independent clauses." He points out that the second major function of a narrative is to establish an evaluative connection between "Event A" and "Event B." Labov states, "Most adult narratives are more than a simple reporting of events. A variety of evaluative devices are used to establish the evaluative point of the story" (Labov 2010: 547). Labov's linguistic analysis is consistent with the cognitive abilities of humans as described by Tomasello. Both Labov and Tomasello emphasize the ability to convey experience to another human.

Labov further expounds on the structure of narrative, indicating the first clause usually includes the orientation, which identifies the participants in the action, the time, the place, and so forth. Labov expands the definition of narrative by saying the evaluative function reports the "So what?" portion of a communication, something that "provides justification for the narrative's claim on a greater portion of conversational time" (Labov 2010: 547), which is another way of saying that narrative may be of mutual interest to conspecifics, one of the fundamental building blocks of cultural meaning. Labov describes this as "reportability or tellability" of an event. The "So what?" or reportability is what connects both the teller and the listener. As I will demonstrate, a diagnosis narrative has a teller and listener – the doctor and the patient. The claim to reportability between the doctor and the patient is the threat of disease and death.

Developing the concept of narrative further, Labov says, "Narratives include a protagonist, antagonist and third party witnesses," indicating the "self as original author of the narrative and its immediate animator" (Labov 2010: 548). Again, this is consistent with how Tomasello details these actions resulting from natural human growth and development beginning at an early age.

Embedded within Labov's definitional structure of narrative is the concept of self; similar to Tomasello, it creates evidence the self exists; the *self narrates*. Labov collected data about the interactions between two individual selves, the narrator and the listener. In the context of a clinical interaction, it is important to keep in mind that the doctor-patient relationship includes two "selves." A clinical encounter is a conversation where these two selves take turns in a conversation.

The two structural functions of narrative are (1) referential and (2) evaluative. The temporal sequence of the narrative, one of the important defining properties, proceeds from the referential function, which allows a recapitulation of experience. The second necessary requirement in the structure of narrative is the evaluative component. In summary, both Tomasello and Labov report extremely concordant results from two distinctly different data sets. Tomasello uses primate interactions and observations of primates while Labov uses observations of linguistic encounters. Together they form the basis for narrative as I explore its cultural dimensions.

Narrative, schema, and self

Roy D'Andrade gives a history of the development of cognitive anthropology and he is closely associated with describing schema theory (1995). He notes that "the schema is an organized framework of objects and relations which has yet to be filled in with concrete details" (D'Andrade 1995: 124).

He also notes that simple schemas are embedded in more complex schemas and that the complexity of human thought is explained with this concept (1995: 124). Using the basic cognitive building blocks of Tomasello and the structure of narrative by Labov, it seems a natural extension that the causal and intentional understanding of human behavior and the description of experience with evaluative function can be combined and expanded into narrative schemas. Cognitive schemas are based on experience. This is consistent with Tomasello's description of human growth and development. D'Andrade presents a small section on consciousness and a discussion of the self:

> The conscious, perceiving center of awareness and agency is the self. . . . It is composed of both the conscious, aware perceiver of the thing that is perceived as doing the perceiving. William James called the perceiver the "I," and the entity perceived the "me." The perceiving self not only observes things in the world, it also perceives that it is perceiving – that is, it is conscious. The perceiving self has a continuing identity through time; it knows that it is the same perceiving self that it was aware of across previous observations – it observes that is the same observer that was observing before.
>
> (D'Andrade 1995: 163)

He goes on to cite evidence that while non-Western models of the mind are not identical to the Western model, there are many commonalities. He quotes Wierzbicka:

> Findings of cross linguistic semantic investigation show that much of the [Western] folk model . . . corresponds in fact to the folk model operating in any other culture of the world: despite the very considerable difference between different folk psychologies that have been described in the literature, the idea of a "person" who "thinks," "wants," "feels," and "knows" (as well as "says" and "does" various things) appears to be universal. The fact that all languages appeared to have words for all of these concepts (though not for "believe" or "desire," as distinct from "think" and "want") provides evidence for the universality of this model.
>
> (Wierzbicka 1993 quoted in D'Andrade 1995: 166)

Relating this to narrative theory, I recognize consensus among these anthropologists that narrative reflects experience of the narrator and that the ability to tell a narrative arises from the interaction of the individual with conspecifics in the cultural environment. Early childhood growth and development provide the basic cognitive framework to engage with human experience, indicating that the biological human being is receptive to developing into a unique individual self. An interactive cycle between being, experience of both interior and external environments as perceived by the individual, generation of narratives related to prior experience, communicating to a conspecific, which then becomes a repeating cycle, has been described. This description supports my claim that he individual self and culture are co-constituent of each other, a distinction from cultural determinism.

The self in culture

Clifford Geertz summarizes the relationship of self to culture as follows: "Becoming human is becoming individual, and we become individual under the guidance of cultural patterns, historically created systems of meaning in terms of which we give form, order, point and direction to our lives" (Geertz 1973: 52).

The cognitive psychologist Jerome Bruner argues that narrative forms experience, but later provides an example where a "perceiving self" developmentally predates the ability to construct a narrative. He thereby argues that experience forms narrative and narrative forms experience – two sides of the same coin. Adopting this paradox is an elegant way of resolving many arguments related to narrative healing. Bruner gives two powerful examples, highlighting these contrasting views. The first is the exodus from Nazi-dominated Europe after the outbreak of World War II and his observations of

> heartbroken people on the boat – families separating for safety, and merchants leaving their businesses behind, refugees fleeing the Nazis – I couldn't help being amused by the ever-ready impulse to see life as imitating art. And I, too, was using the narrative in conceiving that journey: the Shawnee's voyage as yet another enactment of the biblical book of Exodus!
>
> (Bruner 2002: 7)

In that example, Bruner understands his personal experience through a pre-existing narrative, structuring, filtering, and organizing his experience to fit a recognizable story.

Later he talks about audio recordings of an infant while she was alone in bed before she fell asleep:

> She seemed drawn to the unexpected, to things that had surprised her or caught her unprepared. These little surprises would start her off on comments about how she had coped with their likes in the past or would cope with them tomorrow. So intent was she on getting her stories right that we came to believe her progress in acquiring language was driven by some sort of narrative energy. In some way, Emmy seemed to know what a story required for its telling even before she had the grammar needed to tell it right. It was as if a narrative sensibility were guiding her search for the right syntactic forms.
>
> (Bruner 2002: 32)

In retelling the story of Emmy, although not directly referential to the work of Tomasello, his description is perfectly consistent with the theory of the mind as expounded by Tomasello. How Emmy "would cope with them tomorrow" is an example of an intentional and causal self. The goal direction described by Tomasello is the "narrative energy" to overcome the unexpected.

Bruner goes on to say:

> Self making is a narrative art, though it is more constrained by memory than fiction is, it is uneasily constrained, a matter to which we shall come presently. Self making, anomalously, is from both inside and the outside. The inside of it we like to see in our Cartesian way, is memory, feelings, ideas, beliefs, subjectivity. Part of this insidedness is almost certainly innate and species specific, like our irresistible sense of continuity over time and place in our pastoral sense of ourselves. But much of self making is from outside in – based on the apparent esteem of others and on the myriad expectations that we early, even mindlessly pick up from culture in which we are immersed.
>
>   Besides, narrative acts of self making are usually guided by unspoken, implicit cultural models of what selfhood should be, might be – and, of course what shouldn't be . . . Telling others about oneself is, then no simple matter. It depends on what we think they think we ought to be like – or what selves in general ought to be like.
>
> (Bruner 2002: 65–66)

In that passage, Bruner acknowledges the "innate and species specific" attribute of self with characteristics the human capacity to narrate. Additionally, he outlines the cultural influences on that same self:

> None of this seems to discourage us. We go on, constructing ourselves through narrative. Why is narrative so essential, why do we need it for self definition? The narrative gift seems to be our natural way of using language for characterizing those deviations from the expected state of things that characterize living in human culture. None of us knows the just so evolutionary story of its rise and survival. But what we do know is that it is irresistible as a way of making sense of human interaction.
>
> (Bruner 2002: 85)

Based on the foundational aspects of narrative reviewed so far, it is my opinion that the intentional self as described by Tomasello is part of the biological, neurological form of a human. I agree with Geertz when he says, "We are, in sum, incomplete or unfinished animals who complete or finish ourselves through culture – and not to culture in general but through highly particular forms" (Geertz 1973: 49). In this way, there is bidirectional cultural flow between the individual and the cultural body. Although I can accept in part the constructivist perspective of the self, I reject the extreme that there is nothing beyond that. As Tomasello points out, innovation (by a self) is required for participatory learning and the ratchet effect. Each human is in the process of living and experiencing, creating a unique self.

Quoting Strawson in *The Self in Health and Illness*, edited by Frances Rapport and Paul Wainwright, the editors recount:

> By "self-experience," then, I mean the experience that people have of themselves as being, specifically, a mental presence; a mental someone; a single mental something or other. Such self-experience comes to every normal human being, in some form, in early childhood. The realization of the fact that one's thoughts are unobservable by others, the experience of the sense in which one is alone in one's head or mind, the mere awareness of oneself as thinking: these are among the very deepest facts about the character of human life.
>
> (Rapport and Wainwright 2006: 3)

Again, Strawson describes experience as self-experience in relationship with the social environment. The role of self to narrative is definitional.

Cheryl Mattingly has an entire chapter named "The Self in Narrative Suspense: Therapeutic Plots and Life Stories" (1988: 104–128). She contrasts the meaning of life with uncertainty of life and indicates how life plots and therapeutic plots are irrevocably intertwined. She reviews the history of the self in anthropology, citing Mauss, Carrithers, Csordas, and others. Admitting that this is beyond the scope of her book, she summarizes the difficulties anthropologists have had with the concept of self, "the internal private self and a culturally constructed, socially governed public persona" (Mattingly 1998: 105). Unfortunately, she subsequently confounds the term self with person, and discusses the perplexity of the topic, perhaps reflective of the confusion within the discipline of anthropology itself:

> And a dualistic self is provided narrative with confused and even paradoxical place in anthropological thought. Sometimes narrative is linked to publicly knowable self, a cultural or scripted person who could be distinguished from a private, inaccessible inner self. But scholars have also recently turned personal narrative to explore informants sense of self as this relates to, or contrasts with culturally shared meanings. Anthropologists have been drawn to the study of the self as characterized by emotions, personal histories, unique experiences, private ruminations, tacit knowledge, even the unsaid. Here, narrative emerges as a vehicle for exploring just that inner experienced self Geertz (and many others) have declared out of bounds to the anthropologist.
>
> (Mattingly 1998: 105)

Mattingly's word choice includes both "self" with "person." Again, for the purposes of my research, I assert they are theoretically different. For the purposes of clarity, I contend it is the *person* who participates in a public ritual, but it is the *self* that is healed. Mattingly writes:

> On the one hand narrative is elevated to the very thing which guarantees us the ability to have a self, at least in the sense of something we perceived as a unified and whole. On the other, it turns out to be a kind of trickster, a rhetorical ploy by which we disguise the genuine nature of ourselves – as splintered and discontinuous.
>
> (Mattingly 1998: 105–106)

She goes on to state:

> For if narrative helps make an inner phenomenological self coherent, this suggests that there exists a pre-narrated self which is, in its primal state not coherent. This inner self as something experienced is very often depicted as fractured, . . . The coherent self emerges conceptually as an "illusion," a "fiction" which is part of our Western ideology but is not borne out in the individual experience.
>
> (Mattingly 1998: 106)

I find a logical flaw in this statement. Previous theorists have portrayed the self as emergent, making the pre-narrated self *latent*, not *inchoate*. Mattingly reviews all the previous arguments and eventually resorts to philosophy. She summarizes by saying that narrative is often perceived as the prime strategy by which the meaning of life-altering ailment – in the meaning of a life – is created. She acknowledges that narrative deals with breaches of cultural convention (another example of disruption, which I refer to as the existential threat to the self by disease and death).

Narrative and emotions

The discussion of emotion in anthropology is extensive; I will highlight only certain aspects that further the theoretical argument of this research. Alexander Hinton in his introduction to *Biocultural Approaches to the Emotions* (1999) gives one of the first and important reasons to include emotion in the study of narrative. He states, "Emotions are cognitive appraisals that are made and acted upon within an interpersonal social context and on the basis of a culturally relative set of beliefs and values" (Hinton 1999: 8). It is the appraisal or evaluative component of the emotions that is fundamental to Labov's definition of narrative. Hinton widens Labov's evaluation of the relationship between two experiences in the past to evaluating the self in relationship to the world. This draws on themes of self-creation through interaction with experiences of living in the world. Hinton is merely stating that emotions are powerful social tools to accomplish that evaluation.

Carol Worthman, in *Emotions: You Can Feel the Difference* (1999), presents material that is concordant with Bruner. Bruner pointed out that there is an iterative cycle between an individual telling a narrative and a narrative informing the individual's experience and retelling of that experience. This conceptual framework supports the understanding that the individual self and culture are mutually interactive, echoing Geertz's statement. Worthman states:

> Emotions are particularly thorny for anthropologists because they require integration of the individual and cultural levels of explanation, but they are interesting for just that reason. Emotions involve relational-evaluative stances of the individual to situation. Moreover, they effect a crucial link in embodiment of the experiential self by entraining physical states with both individual experience and behavior.
>
> (Worthman 1999: 53)

This statement highlights the evaluative nature of emotions while recognizing the bidirectionality of an emotion between an individual and the cultural body. She draws on other theorists in making this argument, stating:

> Contemporary culture theory increasingly employs the notion of embodiment, a concept initially advanced by Merleau-Ponty (Merleau-Ponty 1962) to indicate this situated-projective relationship of subject to object in perception, and by Bourdieu (Bordieu 1977) to denote the "socially informed body." Conceptions of embodiment address the persistent conceptual gaps between mind and body, individual and society in both social and cognitive theory.
>
> (Worthman 1999: 51)

Restating that argument after diagramming the bidirectional nature of emotions, Worthman says, "Emotions are central to reciprocal processes of bringing forward physical states into personal experience and social behavior, as well as transducing individual social experience into physical states. This dual embodiment instantiates the relationship of individual to culture" (Worthman 1999: 63). Again, the intent is not to have a detailed explanation of emotions and anthropology but to understand the relationship of emotions to narrative. The following statement sets up this argument: "Finally, emotions participate, often crucially and definitively, in meaning making" (Worthman 1999: 49).

Daniel Fessler (1999), in his chapter "Toward an Understanding of the Universality of Second Order Emotions," integrates the Malay emotion *malu* as a socially engaged emotion. *Malu* is described as (1) averted gaze, (2) face turned down and away from others, (3) stooped shoulders, (4) shrinking posture, (5) bent-knee, shuffling gait, (6) reddening of the face and neck, and (7) attempts to avoid being seen, culminating in flight (1999: 84). *Malu* approximates shame in Western culture. These observations occurred in the Malay population. The importance is that Fessler directly supports Tomasello's theory of the mind by placing *malu* in the following social structure:

If   (1) Ego can recall emotions that she experienced in the past,

And   (2) Ego is sufficiently aware of her own actions to make a connection between her emotion displays and the emotion displays of others,

And   (3) Ego is aware that others have minds like our own,

Then   (4) Ego is likely to recognize emotion displays not simply as threatening or rewarding stimuli in the environment, but rather as clues to the internal state of the Other. The clues which displays provide are interpreted on the basis of empathy, the formation of an association between the Other's display and Ego's memory of the subjective experience of the corresponding emotion.

(Fessler 1999: 91)

This bridges the understanding of emotion away from something experienced internally by individual humans to a socially engaged cognition. Fessler details the shared cognition of emotions and broadens our understanding of the theory of the mind. Emotions not only help serve in the evaluative function of telling a narrative, but also contribute to the social learning necessary for the "ratchet effect" described by Tomasello.

Emotions and ritual healing

In *Affecting Experience: Toward a Biocultural Model of Human Emotion*, Keith McNeal continues the conversation on emotion and offers the following comment: "The human perceptual apparatus continually evaluates the status of the organism in its socio-ecological niche, so affective feeling states are implicated in the overall orientational processes of maintaining the organism's well-being in relation to its milieu" (McNeal 1999: 216). He goes through detailed analysis of neuro-anatomy and neurophysiology, constructing a biological model of emotional appraisal. I included his comments in this theoretical discussion because one of his examples closely approximates the thesis of this research. He says:

Consider further the importance of interpretation for the processes of ritual healing and contemporary psychotherapy (Csordas 1994; Frank and Frank 1991; Kleinmann 1988). Kleinman has highlighted the process of evaluative transformation, indicating that successful healing therapies – of whatever sort – are often predicated upon effecting deep changes in the way one knows, and therefore perceives, the world. To a certain extent, this process is one of interpretive reformulation; the problem (anxiety, neurosis, etc.) leading to the healing process can largely emerge as a result of the ways the subject interprets his/her status in the world and then acts upon it. Effective therapy requires a thorough reworking of the patient's problematic, habituated ways of knowing, including reinterpretations of past experience (Lock 1987).

(McNeal 1999: 241)

I explore this discussion of Kleinman's "re-education" or reinterpretations later, not strictly within the context of emotions, but within the context of narrative reinterpretation, acknowledging that narratives include emotions as evaluative components in their basic narrative structure. McNeal discusses emotions and the mutually interactive way in which the self and culture interact. Rather than interpreting narratives, his portrayal is consonant with Tomasello's joint attention and understanding through the other. He also emphasizes the transformative properties of healing rituals. Narratives are also imbued with societal norms, an essential component for meaning making. The concept of the theory of the mind has a strong basis in the biological sciences where the same phenomenon is known as the neuro-anatomy and neurophysiology of *mirror neurons* (Coude et al. 2016).

The need to narrate an existential threat in the clinical encounter

Kleinman first used the term *existential threat* (Kleinman 1988a: 153). This term is also alluded to by W.H.R. Rivers (Rivers 2001 [1924]) and Jerome and Julia Frank (Frank and Frank 1991: 5). I chose to use Kleinman's term "existential threat" not only to refer to disease that threatens to end a life, but also a threat to end the existence of a narrating self. Such a threat causes a strong emotion, resulting in a strong claim of "reportability," to use Labov's term, or a sense of "drama" to use a term that Cheryl Mattingly would use (Mattingly 2000). W.H.R. Rivers first described the threat of disease and death in ritual healing. I combine Rivers's terminology and Kleinman's terminology in a summative way as "*the existential threat of disease and death*." W.H.R. Rivers claims this to be a human universal; I believe this concept touches upon all three bodies – the individual body, the cultural body, and body politic.

I see healing as a broader context than terminal disease – or rather I see each self afflicted not only with a terminal existence manifested with death of the body-self, but also a need of the cultural body to maintain itself in the face of constituent loss.

Bruner introduced the element of the unexpected experience, managed by the telling of a narrative (2002: 32). This unexpected experience foreshadows an essential aspect of what I label the "existential threat of disease" in a clinical encounter. That existential threat calls for a narrative of why it occurred and how to cope with it. Like Emmy, we are self-making creatures, but when the perceiving self is caught in a story of self-unmaking, a story of disease and death, it must cope narratively. No one individual can cope with that alone, so as Tomasello phrases it, we learn through the other. I suggest that humans use a "diagnosis narrative" learned through the other (the doctor) and incorporate that into the schema of the story of the self to navigate the unexpected in life, reclaiming the ability to self-narrate. It is the self, connected to culture through shared narratives, that creates meaning for the individual. Because the narrative is shared, this self is also recognizable to others.

The strong emotions associated with the annihilation of a narrating body-self creates liminality for the individual; the individual can no longer participate fully in culturally defined normative behaviors. The doctor and patient meet in this social space of "anti-structure" and only cultural healing rituals mend the breach. I suggest that when confronted with such a circumstance, the narrating self engages cultural resources of the doctor who draws upon other complex narratives of causal explanations of disease called "diagnosis" to incorporate into one's own self story. I contend that the clinical encounter, with all its narrative and emotional overtones is a process of meaning making. The purpose of this cultural performance is to avert alienation of the diseased individual from the cultural body. Disease alienates; healing reconnects the self with the source of meaning – the cultural body.

Using this theoretical frame, I believe my data show the collaborative interaction of self with culture to deal with the unexpectedness of disease. The existential threat of disease and death is actually a threat to the narrating self.

Healing rituals as narratively structured shared experiences

One of the major discoveries of this research is the relationship of healing rituals to healing relationships. I first explore the "diagnosis narrative," but a diagnosis narrative is really a story within a story. After observing this process hundreds of times, I recognized that "naming the disease" with a narrative story has a rich tradition within the anthropological canon – a healing ritual. Healing rituals are shared experiences with a narrative structure. Cheryl Mattingly highlighted the narrative structure of experience – I extend that concept to the narrative structure of *shared experiences*, described by Tomasello as "learning through the other," which is the part of ritual that I emphasize. This is an important distinction – and a point of departure from other anthropologists. I concentrate on the social practices and performances – NOT the symbolism of ritual. I realize biomedicine is merely a different set of symbolic interactions compared to other healing systems, but comparative culture is not the focus of this research (Kuriyama 1999; Langford 2002; Lewontin 1991). The healing ritual story presented here has a simple plot: a person faced with the existential threat of disease is thrust into a liminal disrupted social space, cut off from daily life. That person seeks out a healer, who is the only socially authorized entity to enter into that same liminal space. The healer (doctor) creates a diagnostic story that the patient can recognize and accept through the process of joint attention with the healer (doctor) to a diagnostic narrative, and together they journey back to full social life, creating along the way a shared experience that bonds them together. I call that culturally structured bond between the patient and doctor a healing relationship.

I intend to develop the concept of a diagnosis narrative and demonstrate cultural practices of medical surgical encounters in our Western medical setting. I will report findings in a parallel process of participant observation where understandings occur in layers and understandings from a larger contextual frame occur in the middle of research. I started with the theoretical frame in this introduction, but after being in the field, a striking ethnographic hypothesis emerged: "Is this really a healing ritual?" I believe the concept of narrative and shared narrative experience is consonant with ritual process, another form of shared experience. I consider the former a prerequisite of understanding the latter, so I present a discussion of ritual in the middle of the ethnographic data, using it subsequently as a heuristic to validate earlier ethnographic analysis related to the diagnosis narrative and prospectively to confirm the hypothesis.

After completing my fieldwork and analysis, I reviewed Barry Saunders's work *CT Suite: The Work of Diagnosis in the Age of Noninvasive Cutting* (Saunders 2008). In many ways, the focus of using computed tomography (CT) images is confirmatory. Thus, Saunders's work and mine are concordant, but differ in intent. We both talk about cultural practices – he describes radiologic film and I describe picture archiving and communication systems (PACS).[1] He talks about *diagnostic rituals*, whereas I talk about *healing rituals*. The patient is practically absent from his work, whereas I try to portray the patient as an active participant in the narratively constructed conversation described by Labov. We use dramatically different theoretical frames; Saunders reinforces power structures and I describe shared experiences where doctors distribute medical power via the cultural body, forming healing relationships. We each inform the others' work.

The self as narrator of self-transformation

Drawing on Kleinman and ritual, McNeal emphasizes the transformative powers of healing rituals as a reworking of the ways of knowing and of experiences. In this way, a narrating self is a transforming self; in a simplistic way, it is a form of lifelong growth and development.

Naomi Quinn reinforces the concept of a narrating self as a transforming self and the idea that new ways of knowing change the way we experience our lives. She discusses how cultural schemas are incorporated into the narrating self and "self-understandings." She directly relates self-understandings to existential concerns. Quinn states:

> If "self-understandings" are more than a semantic gloss for "general goal schemas," then the substitution must hold some new implication. I believe that it does. We are now led to ask, what is it about self-understanding that is so compelling to us that it defines our most general

goals? The answer lies in the way we come to understand ourselves. The process by which cultural schemas are incorporated into a sense of "self," thereby entering into the definition of an individual's existential concerns and life ambitions, is lifelong and causally complex. Most of us would agree that crucial stages of this process of self-definition is occurring in childhood and adolescence; however, dramatic or otherwise compelling experiences at any age can inspire redefinition of the self or elaboration of prior self-understandings.

(Quinn 1992: 91)

Quinn's description approximates a psychological model, but is also consonant with the work of Tomasello. It acknowledges the uniqueness of a self as distinguished from the other while allowing for the evaluative process of experiences and interactions between the two. Tomasello acknowledged that conflicting or differing understandings of the self from attributions of others are possible and it is the interaction of the individual human being with the environment, including the social environment, where the bootstrapping process of creating a self-narrative begins.

Quinn's description is also consistent with the model of ritual healing and healing relationships presented in this research. She outlines an anthropology of the self that is entirely consistent with McNeal and is a model that I highly endorse. This particular passage is almost an anthropological description of psychotherapy. Because of the metonymic use of "existential concerns" and "self-understandings," I connect her work with what I will later describe as the appropriate setting for Kleinman's illness narratives. My major argument is that such existential concerns of the self are part of routine clinical encounters. I will make this same argument when discussing clinical encounters as narratively structured rituals.

A word of caution about conflated anthropological taxonomies

In the preceding discussion, I chose anthropological theorists that are consistent with my own beliefs. I have also read the work of other anthropologists whose work have gained wide acceptance but whose work lacks face validity from my perspective. For the purposes of disclosure, I present their work to indicate why I do not find their work practical or useful.

Robert Hahn, in his book, *Sickness and Healing: An Anthropological Perspective*, claims to widen anthropological perspectives. He states, "Broadly speaking, the essence of 'sickness' is an unwanted condition in one's person or self – one's mind, body, soul, or connection to the world" (Hahn 1995: 5). He goes on to state:

It is not commonly recognized in the West that ideas about what a "person" and "self" are and should be differ greatly from one cultural setting to another. Indeed, the individual weighted person, separate from the rest of society in the universe, is a distinctly Western notion (Dumont 1965; Lutz 1985); in many non-Western societies, persons are regarded as essentially an inextricably linked with other beings, human and nonhuman. Autonomy and independence are also largely Western values about desirable connection with others.

(Hahn 1995: 5)

This statement echoes that more famous reference by Geertz:

But at least some conception of what human individual is, as opposed to a rock, and animal, a rainstorm, or a god, is, as far as I can see, universal. Yet at the same time, as these offhand examples suggest, the actual conceptions involved vary from one group to the next, and often quite sharply. The Western conception of the person as a bounded, unique, more or less integrated motivational and cognitive universe, a dynamic center of awareness, emotion, judgment, and action organized into a distinctive whole and set contrastively both against other such wholes and against its social and natural background, is, however incorrigible it may seem to us, a rather peculiar idea within the context of world cultures.

(Geertz 1984: 126)

I struggled with both Hahn's and Geertz's pronouncements for years and finally came to reject them. My prior discussion of a narrating self provides a contrasting formulation to their statements. Up to this point, I have used the terms *individual* and *self*, avoiding the term *person*. The question immediately becomes, "What is the anthropological relationship between person and self?" Reviewing Hahn's definition of sickness, he conflates person and self and lists attributes of that entity as mind, body, soul, or connection to the world (1995: 5). I believe these are conflated terms leading to false dichotomies and not helpful for this research. *I contend that within the context of this research, person is a cultural construction and, as such, a cultural actor responsive to external expectations of socially appropriate behavior. Self is a cognitive component of an individual, unique in the sense that Tomasello points out, who may choose to incorporate what it perceives in the cultural environment or choose to reject it.*

My simplistic formulation of distinguishing self from person and using self as the context of this research avoids the philosophical and scholarly debates regarding the object of healing. This surprises even me, as I had previously differentiated "curing disease" from "healing the person." I now believe that the person, as a cultural construction, is not universally the same in all cultures; the self, however, is a universal. I contend that the enduring and transforming self is the object of healing and the self is the anthropological entity that defines a healing relationship within the cultural body. I define *illness narratives* as stories told by persons acting as social actors. I define *healing relationships* as shared experience between two selves. Although others may criticize my nomenclature as overly simplistic, I use it as a corrective response to anthropological literature that is conflated and less helpful for this research project because it expands the scope of the argument to the point that it is no longer manageable.

If I were to put the controversies into context, I would say Geertz and Hahn have "hypo-cognitivized" the self in the sense that Levy describes certain emotions in certain cultures as hypo-cognitivized (Levy 1984: 219). Just because they are hard to observe or may not be expressed by members of the culture is not the equivalent to nonexistence. I mention this here to caution the reader about conflated terms. As I present data, results, and analysis, I will emphasize the words *individual self, illness*, and *disease*, as they lend themselves to a more parsimonious argument. Scheper-Hughes and Lock used the term "individual body-self," a term much closer to the theoretical underpinnings of this research study (1987: 1).

Arthur Kleinman and Cheryl Mattingly both have a corpus of anthropological work directly related to narrative and culture; both of them conflate person and self, at times using them interchangeably. Yet both acknowledge the clinical encounter as a healing ritual. In this research, I discuss both healing rituals and healing relationships. I intend to show that healing rituals allow the development of healing relationships. For the purposes of clarity in argument, I will define someone who participates in a ritual as a *person* and define someone who is part of a healing relationship as a *self*, a self that has incorporated the *other* into a self-narrative. Clarifying this ambiguity is essential to sorting through all the conflicting literature on the topic of healing.

A guide to the organization of data presentation

Nancy Scheper-Hughes and Margaret Lock described this relationship between the self and society in their landmark paper (Scheper-Hughes and Lock 1987). I believe that anthropological research should use the "triangulation" of self, culture, and body politic to demonstrate validity of the research project. For this reason, I present the ethnographic data in this format, using "the three bodies." In addition to providing validity, "the three bodies" heuristic is fundamental to understanding the relationship of the self to society. Based on Tomasello's work, I believe culture would not exist in the absence of a human self; likewise, the human self would not survive without culture.

Note

1 The PACS system figures prominently in the ethnographic data I present. Essentially, there are two computer systems with differing functions. A CT scan is a two-dimensional image generated by a computer from multiple linear data points. The second computer system is the PACS system, which allows the images to be viewed over a network distributed in time and space.

References

Bourdieu, Pierre. 1977. *Outline of a Theory of Practice*. Cambridge: Cambridge University Press.

Bruner, Jerome. 2002. *Making Stories: Law, Literature, and Life*. New York: Farrar, Straus and Giroux.

Coude, Gino, et al. 2016. Mirror Neurons of Ventral Premotor Cortex Are Modulated by Social Cues Provided by Others' Gaze. *Journal of Neuroscience* 36(11).

Csordas, Thomas. 1994. *The Sacred Self: A Cultural Phenomenology of Charismatic Healing*. Berkeley: University of California Press.

D'Andrade, Roy. 1995. *The Development of Cognitive Anthropology*. New York: Cambridge University Press.

Dumont, Louis. 1965. The Modern Conception of the Individual: Notes on Its Genesis. *Contributions to Indian Sociology* 8:13–61.

Fessler, Daniel. 1999. Toward an Understanding of the Universality of Second Order Emotions. *In Biocultural Approaches to the Emotions*. A.L. Hinton, ed. Cambridge: Cambridge University Press.

Frank, Jerome D., and Julia B. Frank. 1991. *Persuasion & Healing: A Comparative Study of Psychotherapy*. Baltimore: Johns Hopkins University Press.

Geertz, Clifford. 1973. *The Interpretation of Cultures*. New York: Basic Books.

———. 1984. On the Nature of Anthropological Understanding. *In Culture Theory: Essays on Mind, Self, and Emotion*. R. Shweder and R. Levine, eds. Cambridge: Cambridge University Press.

Hahn, Robert A. 1995. *Sickness and Healing*. New Haven, CT: Yale University Press.

Hinton, Alexander Laban. 1999. Introduction: Developing a biocultural approach to the emotions. *In Biocultural Approaches to the Emotions*. A.L. Hinton, ed. Cambridge: Cambridge University Press.

Kleinman, Arthur. 1988a. *The Illness Narratives – Suffering, Healing, and the Human Condition*. New York: Basic Books.

———. 1988b. *Rethinking Psychiatry: From Cultural Category to Personal Experience*. New York: Free Press.

Kuriyama, Shigehisa. 1999. *The Expressiveness of the Body: and the Divergence of Greek and Chinese Medicine*. Brooklyn: Zone Books.

Labov, William. 2010. Narratives of Personal Experience. *In Cambridge Encyclopedia of the Language Sciences*. P. Hogan, ed. Cambridge: Cambridge University Press.

Langford, Jean M. 2002. *Fluent Bodies: Ayurvedic Remedies for Postcolonial Imbalance*. Durham, NC: Duke University Press.

Levy, Robert I. 1984. Emotion, Knowing, and Culture. *In Culture Theory: Essays on Mind, Self, and Emotion*. R.A. Shweder and R.A. LeVine, eds. Pp. 88–119. Cambridge: Cambridge University Press.

Lewontin, Richard C. 1991. *Biology as Ideology: The Doctrine of DNA*. New York: HarperCollins.

Lock, Margaret. 1987. DSM-III as a Culture-Bound Construct: Commentary on Culture-Bound Syndromes and International Disease Classification. *Culture, Medicine, and Psychiatry* 11:35–42.

Lutz, Cathereine. 1985. Ethnopsychology Compared to What? Explaining Behavior and Consciousness Among the Ifaluk. *In Person, Self, and Experience*. G.M. White and J. Kirkpatrick, eds. Berkeley: University of California Press.

Mattingly, Cheryl. 1998. *Healing Dramas and Clinical Plots: The Narrative Structure of Experience*. Cambridge: Cambridge University Press.

———. 2000. Emergent Narratives. *In Narrative and the Cultural Construction of Illness and Healing*. C. Mattingly and L. C. Garro, eds. Pp. 181–211. Berkeley: University of California Press.

McNeal, Keith E. 1999. Affecting Experience: Toward a Biocultural Model of Human Emotion. *In Biocultural Approaches to the Emotions*. A. L. Hinton, ed. Cambridge: Cambridge University Press.

Merleau-Ponty, Maurice. 1962. *Phenomenology of Perception*. London: Routledge and Kegan Paul.

Murphey, Keith M., and Jason Throop, eds. 2010. *Toward an Anthropology of the Will*. Stanford: Stanford University Press.

Quinn, Naomi. 1992. The Motivational Force of Self-Understanding: Evidence From Wives' Inner Conflicts. *In Human Motives and Cultural Models*. R. D. Andrade and C. Strauss, eds. Cambridge: Cambridge University Press.

Rapport, Frances, and Paul Wainwright. 2006. Introduction: The Nature of Self and How It Is Experienced Within and Beyond the Healthcare Setting. *In The Self in Health and Illness: Patients, Professionals and Narrative Identity*. F. Rapport and P. Wainwright, eds. Pp. 1–6. Oxford: Radcliffe.

Rivers, W.H.R. 2001 [1924]. *Medicine, Magic, and Religion*. London: Routledge Classics.

Saunders, Barry F. 2008. *CT Suite: The Work of Diagnosis in the Age of Noninvasive Cutting*. Durham, NC: Duke University Press.

Scheper-Hughes, N., and M. M. Lock. 1987. The Mindful Body: A Prolegomenon to Future Work in Medical Anthropology. *Medical Anthropology Quarterly* 1:6–41.

Tomasello, Michael. 1999. *The Cultural Origins of Human Cognition*. Cambridge, MA: Harvard University Press.

Wierzbicka, Anna. 1993. A Conceptual Basis for Cultural Psychology. *ETHOS* 21(2):205–231.

Worthman, Carol M. 1999. Emotions: You Can Feel the Difference. *In Biocultural Approaches to the Emotions*. A. L. Hinton, ed. Pp. 41–74. Cambridge: Cambridge University Press.

Part II
The diagnosis narratives

3 Entrance into the field

The doctor stood staring at the computer screen next to the countertop sink, searching screen after screen, occasionally flipping papers from printed sections of the electronic medical record, pondering, silently lost in thought. The patient sat silently staring at his back; who knew what the patient was thinking? I never heard an illness narrative for the rest of my first day in the field . . . what were all those anthropological textbooks I read about illness narratives talking about? I felt like Stanislaw Malinowski with all my anthropological baggage on the beach, not knowing a thing about what was going on.

First impressions

I started my fieldwork in an outpatient urology office associated with the university. Three urologists shared this office: Dr. Stein, Dr. Jeffries, and Dr. Patel. All three of them saw patients from general urology, but Dr. Patel also had plastic and reconstructive experience, Dr. Stein was a cancer treatment specialist, and Dr. Jeffries had a broad range of patients. Dr. Stein was the chair of the urology department at the university. He was serious, widely published, demonstrated a deep understanding of statistical concepts, and was considered to be the finest robotic urological surgeon in the area. Dr. Jeffries was the urology Residency Program Director. He was jovial, balding with close-cut hair, and always smiling. He was in charge of all the resident physicians who were doing their post-graduate training in urology. Three medical assistants[1] – Marsha, Carmen, and Barbara – worked with the doctors. Occasionally a departmental administrator spent a half-day in the clinic. Between the chair of the department and the Residency Program Director, this was metaphorically the outpatient practice of the chief and the medicine man of the tribe. The name of the office was the Maplewood clinic, across the street from Maplewood Hospital. In many ways, the department and teaching program was like a tribe. I explored the social relationships and culture, following the locales and interactions of this practice, as if it was a tightly defined fieldwork site – the village.

My earliest observations started with one of the medical assistants, Marsha, calling the patient out of the waiting room and bringing him back into an exam room in the clinic. She referred to this process as "rooming a patient." The physical setup is standardized for all the exam rooms, with the exam table underneath the window that spanned from sidewall to sidewall on the top half of the room on the opposite side from the door. The chair for the patient was against the wall between the exam table and the countertop with the sink and the computer. A curtain hanging from a semi-circular ceiling track could be pulled to conceal the exam table if needed. All nine of the exam rooms were along a straight corridor after entering the clinic.

Marsha greeted each patient; she took the patient's blood pressure with an automated blood pressure cuff. She then turned around and typed the vital signs and medical updates into the computer while asking further routine questions while still facing the computer with her back turned to the patient. This means she asked the questions and, hearing the patient's voice from behind her, directly entered the information into the computer program. There was minimal to no eye contact during this part of "rooming the patient." Marsha asked, "Have there been any changes in your medications, your pharmacy, or any changes in allergies? Why are you here today? Are you doing well?" Without sitting down, she typed each response into the computerized medical record using the keyboard of the computer standing on the countertop in the exam room. Sometimes, while eliciting the complaint she started verbally administering the American Urological Association Symptom Score.[2] If it was a new patient, she gathered information on the past medical, family, and social history in the same manner, always using triple- or quadruple-barreled questions, sometimes double-triple-barreled questions. "Do your mother-father's siblings have diabetes, hypertension, or cancer?" I watched hundreds of office visits and they all began this same way. My overwhelming first impression was that I was observing a more rigorous form of a structured medical interview similar that described by Elliot Mischler (Mischler 1986: 54–59). In this case, however, it was even more overt – the only allowable responses were those that fit into the database structure of the computerized medical record.

Patients didn't seem to find this unusual or unexpected. In fact, the following example illustrates an extreme case. The patient was new to the clinic, a young African American I estimated to be in his twenties. As mentioned before, the patient sat in the chair next to the exam table after entering the room. This particular patient had an iPhone in his left hand and another smartphone in his right hand. Throughout the entire intake interview by Marsha, the patient was surfing the web, checking text messages, and interacting with his iPhone while Marsha was asking him questions and entering the data into the computer. Both Marsha and the patient focused on a digital device, but this time both were looking away from the other. This example will become important as a contrast to my later findings, but at the time, I was bewildered because this was definitely not an illness narrative.

The patient was actually multitasking, answering medical history questions while surfing the internet with his phones. The presenting complaint was frequent urination, which he had had for years, and the patient reported that he had an InterStim[3] procedure done at Benedict Hospital. The patient characterized it as needles going in his back. I thought he said something about getting the evaluation but never actually having the procedure. Marsha repeated back to him that he had had the procedure done and entered it into the computer as if that were true.

Where is the illness narrative?

Right from the beginning of fieldwork, I recognized the pattern of interaction was not what I had expected. Why have so many anthropologists linked healing with narrative? Where were the illness narratives I had expected? At the time, I had a twinge of ethnocentric judgment of the medical team, echoing the anthropological canon of systematically de-humanizing patients by writing the patient's story as one of disease and not illness. As I observed and understood more, I realized how inaccurate those initial thoughts were. At least I was in a good place to start ethnographic research – officially confused. I wiped my mind clean of preconceived notions and simply observed, trying to understand what was happening during an office visit in a urology clinic.

I found similarities between the medical assistants' process of "rooming a patient" and the senior staff interactions with the patients. Similar to Marsha, Dr. Jeffries radiated happiness and a positive attitude. Yet that didn't translate into eliciting an illness narrative. Upon entering the room on one occasion, Dr. Jeffries almost immediately started asking a pointed series of questions that was a verbal form of the American Urological Association Symptom Score. He ended with the question, "Does this bother you enough to take a medicine?" Both the patient and the patient's wife were sitting there, and after a pause, the patient indicated that he might be interested in it. Dr. Jeffries said, "Your cancer is up to snuff, so now we're focusing on quality-of-life issues." The next section of the interview was part of a standard medical interview called the review of systems. Dr. Jeffries turned his back to the patient and his wife, and asked questions directly off the computer screen and entered the answers in the computer as the patient was answering. The electronic medical record has an underlying database format, so the answers were either yes/no recorded with a toggle button or a series of pre-formatted responses requiring a click of the computer mouse to choose among the options. Both the patient and his wife were observing the back of Dr. Jeffries's head during this interaction. Again, similar to my earlier comment about Mischler's analysis of the medical interview, it seemed as though the computer was asking the questions instead of the doctor. In these examples, the tightly structured interview was a reflection of the software program of the electronic medical record. The absence of an illness narrative was glaringly obvious. I was familiar enough with the software to know that there were no radio buttons in the database for an emotion and being familiar with databases, I knew it was impossible to create a "cause-and-effect" sequence in the computer output. Later, I will point out an example later when Dr. Jeffries comments on these deficiencies.

The next example illustrates a similar process with more complexity. The patient was Chinese and came with a family member as interpreter. The exact relationship between the patient and his translator was never determined. Marsha put them both in the room, then had the patient go to the bathroom and immediately did the urinalysis.[4] Since this was a new patient, she attempted to take a complete history, but he did not know the name of the medicine he was taking and he did not know his pharmacy, at which point Marsha had to turn around and face the patient to try to get information. The patient spoke very few English words, and the interpreter translated most of the interaction.

Marsha asked, "Why are you here?"

"I don't know."

She checked the electronic medical record and asked him, "Do you have a headache or dizziness?"

"Yes."

Marsha said, "Those are neurologic problems, not urologic problems." At this point, Marsha appeared frustrated because she could not determine the reason why his primary care doctor sent him here for consultation. Having acquired no information of value, she left the exam room and started checking the computer on her desktop, saying to herself, "It must be an elevated PSA[5] or voiding problems." It was at this point that she called the primary care doctor's office and scanned through the electronic medical record.

When Marsha went back into the exam room the caregiver for the patient said, "Did you ask if he had it or they said he had it?" The interpreter was referring to a CAT scan.

Marsha said, "He must've had an elevated PSA, and they're checking his prostate level."

The caregiver asked, "Does he have an infection?"

Marsha replied, "It looks like you had an ultrasound, but I don't see a PSA. But based on the size of his prostate, it may be elevated." Marsha continued typing in the electronic health record and then asked, "Is he having trouble voiding,[6] stopping, starting, nighttime voiding, or anything like that?"

An extensive conversation followed, all in Chinese, lasting several minutes. At the conclusion of the conversation, the caregiver turned to Marsha and said, "No." At that point in the conversation, the caregiver asked, "What's the prostate?"

Marsha replied, "It's an organ only men have." Marsha then proceeded to ask about past medical history, family history, cigarette consumption, etc. When she was done, she told the patient and interpreter that Dr. Patel would be in shortly. Dr. Patel was more formal in the exam room and demonstrated the hierarchy so typical of medical practices.

When Dr. Patel entered the room, he asked the patient, "What's the problem?"

The caregiver replied, "We have no idea. He had an ultrasound, but we don't know the results."

Dr. Patel had spent perhaps less than a minute perusing the computer to ascertain that they did not know why the patient was there. He tried to find the referring physician and then he left the room, saying to Marsha, "He doesn't know why he's here. I wonder if it's an increased PSA? It must be a PSA problem."

Marsha replied, "There are 13 pages of medical information in the electronic health record filed under outside records."

At that point, Dr. Patel returned to the exam room and again engaged with the electronic medical record, reading all 13 pages, which included a CT scan and ultrasound, etc. There was dead silence in the room for an extended time while Dr. Patel was reading off the computer screen (with his back turned to the patient and interpreter). Dr. Patel finally broke the silence by saying, "He's here because of microscopic hematuria and an enlarged prostate."

The caregiver then repeated the words "microscopic hematuria" and said, "I tried to find what that was."

Dr. Patel replied, "I found the problem. He needs a test. It's like a telescopic check of the bladder. We're going to check for cancer cells." He then turned to the computer without any further explanation, questions, or examination and started to type into the computer using his two index fingers. He types hunt-and-peck style. During this prolonged interaction with the computer, he answered a telephone call on his iPhone but continued typing. When he was done typing he told the patient to come out into the hallway. Dr. Patel told Marsha the explanation of why the patient was there and said, "Marsha, book him for a cystoscopy on June 1 at 11:30 a.m."

The caregiver asked if the procedure could be done on the Monday instead of a Wednesday and she was told, "No, the schedule won't allow it." Marsha then gave very careful instructions about having to go back to the primary care physician, getting a referral with an authorization number[7] and procedure code[8] on it, and bring that back with them. "If you don't get that referral code, the procedure will be canceled and rescheduled. There should be enough time to get the paperwork completed."

After the office visit, I asked Marsha about her perception of the encounter. She said, "It was hard because getting the patient's personal information was hard work with a translator. I called the primary care doctor's office and got told that there was only one person working there and he didn't have the time to find the ultrasound or provide information about the referral. That slowed down patient flow here."

Carmen (the medical assistant usually teamed up with Dr. Jeffries) interrupted, saying, "I was dumbfounded that a patient would show up without knowing why they were at the doctor's office. The referral process in the healthcare system should be much more careful about having the information available." Carmen expressed this same sentiment several times on other occasions. "This is frustrating. He [the patient] doesn't speak a lick of English. I've looked online for labs and his renal ultrasound – who knows? We call ourselves Sherlock Holmes here; we're always investigating why they're here. I've tried calling the primary care office, and all I got was a message and a phone recording. There's no referral. There's no procedure code. The referral's been cancelled and he's going off on me. Dr. Jeffries already yelled at me."

This office visit demonstrates the fragmented and contradictory nature of the narrative during an office visit. Carmen's characterization of Sherlock Holmes best described the inexplicability of circumstances in the clinic. Of course, each Sherlock Holmes episode written by Arthur Conan Doyle ends with a tight narrative that explains all the incongruent information succinctly. Instead of Sherlock Holmes, it takes an ethnographer doing participant observation to explain what really happened that day. For the time being, I was still "officially confused."

Although confused, I had learned important information. Illness narratives are not part of a clinical office encounter. I have no doubt that they exist, simply not in the social space of a clinical encounter. Although I present something that could be called illness narratives in Appendix A of this book, I believe the methodological distinction caused by interviewing patients compared to participant observation explains the discrepancy. I remember being unable to recall reading ethnographic data collected during a medical surgical clinical office visit and recognized how my confusion was already expanding the ethnographic record of clinical encounters. I surmise that patients tell illness narratives outside the doctor's office, such as when someone asks, "How did it go today at the doctor's office?"

In my personal experience, I listen to many illness narratives in social settings such as at church or at social gatherings – people love to tell their illness stories, both good and bad. This directly contradicts Arthur Kleinman who claimed that the medical healthcare system needed to be reformed, "Legitimating the patient's illness experience – authorizing that experience, auditing it empathically – is a key task in the care of the chronically ill" (Kleinman 1988: 18). Kleinman's comments resonate with others that "healing" is "witnessing to the suffering of the other" (Egnew 2005). As my research proceeded, I discovered a completely different type of witnessing to suffering, making my disagreement with Kleinman one of process, not concept. I actually agree with Kleinman's formulation, but what I discovered in my confusion was that bearing witness to illness narratives is not the norm for clinical encounters, making my own research important because it describes the underreported activity that has a universal formulation of the social practice of healing.

From these initial observations and all of the visits that followed, I concluded that the illness narrative was not a significant part of the outpatient clinical encounter for a new problem, contradicting what I believed throughout my medical and anthropological studies. I couldn't identify the narrator, I couldn't figure out what the story was about, and although I was observing a rigidly structured cultural performance, I didn't know the purpose of the participants' behaviors. I understood then that prior anthropological research had gaps in the data and interpretation of "healing" or "narrative healing." I needed to conceptualize my data differently than others while staying consistent with anthropological enterprise and theory.

Notes

1 A medical assistant is a trained individual and has a certification to perform tasks in medical settings involving patient care and routine clerical jobs.
2 The American Urologic Association Symptom Score (AUASS) is a validated, standardized psychometric exam measuring obstruction to urine flow as experienced by the patient.
3 InterStim is a device made by Medtronic that modulates the nerve stimulation to the bladder, often used to control an overactive bladder, a condition that sometimes leads to leaking of urine.
4 A urinalysis involves dipping a plastic stick into the urine and watching nine different pads soaked with reagents turn colors, each detecting a different property of the urine, such as glucose (sugar), pH (acidity), specific gravity (how many salts and proteins were in dissolved in the urine, and so forth.
5 Prostate-specific antigen (PSA) is a blood test for a specific protein used to screen for prostate cancer or monitor the management of prostate cancer.
6 Voiding means emptying the bladder.
7 An authorization number is an indication of pre-authorization from the health insurance company. This allows the insurance company to review the clinical case before authorizing payment.
8 Current Procedural Terminology (CPT) code is a standardized nomenclature of medical procedures, again allowing authorization for billing of services provided. It is a necessary part of obtaining a referral code.

References

Egnew, Thomas R. 2005. The Meaning of Healing: Transcending Suffering. *Annals of Family Medicine* 3(3):255–263.

Kleinman, Arthur. 1988. *The Illness Narratives – Suffering, Healing, and the Human Condition*. New York: Basic Books.

Mischler, Elliot G. 1986. *Research Interviewing: Context and Narrative*. Cambridge, MA: Harvard University Press.

4 Who is narrating and what story are they telling?

I was familiar with narrative schemas (D'Andrade 1995; Tomasello 1999). I recognized the database structure of the computer program and the American Urological Association Symptom Score (AUASS) as templates – the schemas – to construct the narrative. Although I continued to observe for behaviors of the patient that contributed to this overall narrative, my subsequent observations remained consistent with my experiences that first day of fieldwork. My next question and objective of observations was to locate and identify where the narrative was located and who the *narrator* was. I recognized how important this process was, as illustrated by the following vignette:

> Dr. Jeffries told the patient, "I can't get a copy of your MRI to figure out if the [kidney] stone is still present. I wouldn't be doing you any favors if I took the stent[1] out if the stone was still there. That's why this information is essential." Dr. Jeffries left the exam room and asked Carmen, "They are supposed to be sending it, aren't they?"
> "Yes."
> Dr. Jeffries said, "If we need to call again, I will call Regent's Hospital. If I call, I'll make people jump."
> Carmen went into the exam room and came back out saying, "I got the phone number."
> Dr. Jeffries repeated, "I don't have a CT scan, but we need the results so we can take out his stent today."

I had timed the entire process of tracing the CT or MRI data, recording over an hour delay for Carmen, Dr. Jeffries, and the patient. To use Carmen's words, this type of investigation, Sherlock Holmes–style, was a frustration. I called this balance of identifying what data the doctor needed and how to acquire it "collecting the narrative elements." Narrative elements are the details that embody the skeleton of narrative schemas. At this point, I had no idea what the story was about, but I recognized the importance of the process to the experience for all involved. I was beginning to get the sense that the narrative schema called for the doctor to be the narrator of the diagnosis – counterintuitive, but complementary to the assumption that the patient was the narrator of the illness. This became a consistent theme throughout the research.

More examples of narrative schemas – assembling the diagnosis narrative

At this point, I was still observing to locate the narrative. The following example confirms the diagnosis is a narrative schema, and one of the roles of the doctor, together with the office staff, is to collect narrative elements.

When doctors work together, the process becomes easier to observe, as they have to confirm verbally with each other the cognitive components of the diagnosis narrative. Because the doctors engage in a shared social practice, I was able to observe it. Consider the following clinical encounter and note that filling in the narrative schema takes precedence over the actual experience of the patient, again confirming that the illness narrative is not a component of the diagnosis narrative, even though the patient may be the source of part of the data.

Dr. Stein gave Dr. Williamson[2] specific instructions to make sure he read the self-administered history and physical questionnaire before going in to see the patient. When entering the room, Dr. Williamson asked only one open-ended question, which began, "Can you tell me about . . ."

The patient used English as a second language, and his expressive ability was limited. He said, "I am not going through my urine – not strong. I'm worried that there might be something wrong." Later in the interview, the patient asked, "Did a kidney stone get into my prostate and that's what is causing the problem?"

Dr. Williamson was nodding and occasionally said, "Sure," inadvertently responding "yes" to the patient's concern. Without a transition, Dr. Williamson started asking standardized questions, "How long have you had these symptoms? When did you have the stone? Is there any burning when you urinate? Do you wake up in the night to urinate?" The patient apologized because his English wasn't very good. Dr. Williamson said, "You left out a couple of answers here [on the self-administered form]." Dr. Williamson brought the rolling seat (a stool) closer to the patient and directed the patient's attention to the paper.

The patient said, "I didn't understand the question."

Dr. Williamson rephrased some of the questions (going over the AUASS) and after talking to the patient without being able to ascertain the patient's answer, said, "We will just say less than one in five."

At that point, the patient said, "I can hold my urine but it is painful to do it." At that point, I noticed that Dr. Williamson checked the lowest score for that item on the AUASS.[3]

Dr. Williamson went out of the exam room to present the case to Dr. Stein, who asked about the PSA. Dr. Williamson just said, "The patient said his doctor checked it and it was okay."

Interjecting, Dr. Jeffries leaned over and said, "Did you check here?" indicating the computer.

Dr. Williamson went on presenting the case to Dr. Stein and said, "The prostate is 30 grams with a good medial sulcus.[4] The patient scored 6 on the AUASS, but he was not satisfied."

Dr. Stein said, "Did you give him all the adjectives?"

"Yes, I did."

Dr. Stein said, "Happy, not happy," and proceeded to list five or six more possible adjectives.[5]

Dr. Williamson said, "He's not pleased."

Dr. Stein said, "Google it [AUASS] and you can get it in two seconds – I'm old, you're young." It seemed at the time that Dr. Stein wanted a thorough, accurate, and complete American Urological Association Symptom Score recorded in the chart. His questions about "happy" was pure sarcasm because that type of question does not appear on the AUASS.

This vignette is similar to the earlier one in that there was a language barrier; the patient was not the source of the necessary narrative elements. Doctors will fill in a medical history template, even if they have to interpolate or guess at the answers. Important at this point in the investigation, I became aware of how many different scattered sources the narrative elements came from. I also recognized how important collecting such data was.

The doctor is heavily dependent upon a team of personnel to collect the data. In the scenarios presented in this chapter, I am trying to illustrate that variety; the data are the narrative components. Not only are ancillary personnel necessary for the doctor to function, but the data collection starts and ends by inputting and extracting data from the computer. In this manner, computer networks are the keepers of the narrative elements as many different, widespread sources input data. This constitutes a distributed cognitive network similar to that described by Edwin Hutchins (1995). Doctors, like engineers, rely on data to function in their job. Current practice requires a complete dataset that needs to be acquired, stored, interpreted, and rearchived, awaiting the doctor to formulate and speak the "diagnostic narrative." I present several examples to illustrate this point.

One day I walked into the clinic and it was immediately apparent that Carmen and Dr. Jeffries were having trouble accessing clinical data. The computer system had crashed. Dr. Jeffries asked Carmen, "Have we asked if they could print it and fax it, because we can't do a thing until I get them?" The administrator at the office was simultaneously talking to someone downtown in administration, recognizing that difficulty accessing the information would disrupt the entire clinic schedule and cause patient dissatisfaction.

Carmen called the IT [Information Technology] help desk and said, "My boss was talking to someone downtown, and they're going to print it and fax it over to us." By saying this, she was acknowledging that the computer system downtown was unable to make the electronic records available at the Maplewood clinic. On similar occasions, I recorded the time that Carmen spent doing this type of work, and it occasionally took her over an hour to get a specific report or piece of clinical data.

"I can't do a thing until we get them," is a revealing statement. Here Dr. Jeffries is saying that he cannot function in the basic role of the doctor unless he can access the data that is ordinarily stored in the computer. What was Dr. Jeffries supposed to do? From an anthropological perspective, I have labeled the database elements and computerized images "narrative elements." What the medical team was struggling to do was obtain the basic narrative elements or components described by Labov – Event A and Event B with an evaluative relationship that supports a cause-and-effect telling of experience. Dr. Jeffries is supposed to combine those narrative elements with a narrative schema to be able to formulate and tell a narrative – a diagnostic narrative. A diagnostic narrative was not what I was expecting to find, but these episodes led me to the ethnographic hypothesis that I had at least found a "narrative," although one that has never been described in such a way. "Narrative medicine" has always been described from the patients' perspective. Often, the imposition of a biomedical label is described as something foreign that patients don't recognize and has been characterized by social scientists as a form of oppression (Foucault 1973, 1994; Frank 1995) or "anti-narrative speech" (Mattingly 1998). I find these descriptions incorrect. If anything, a diagnostic narrative is a complementary narrative act – it simply occurs in a different social space.

Having found a narrative during an outpatient office visit, I used this as an anchor to organize my observations related to other behaviors of the medical assistants, the doctors, and the patients. I believed this was ethnographically appropriate because tremendous amount of time and energy was spent on the process – it was the single most important task of the clinical team. The doctors and medical assistants did all of this work outside in the hallways, out of sight of the patients. It was almost always done prior to ever greeting the patient for the office visit. I started expecting to find illness narratives, but slowly realized I was observing diagnostic narratives, a profound realization. I did not yet know the significance or why it was so important, but I realized it was the work of the doctor. The interaction with the patient is yet to be described.

As I continued to observe, I paid particular attention to what type of data was stored in the computer and how the doctor used that data. The following demonstrates this same point:

> Dr. Jeffries's last patient of the day had kidney stones, and he told me she declined any type of metabolic workup. As we entered the room, he confirmed that was her decision. The patient said, "I doesn't want to take pills."
>
> Dr. Jeffries then proceeded to give a long list of precautions, such as drinking copious amounts of water to keep the urine dilute, avoiding certain food, etc. The patient listened patiently and then replied, "I'm already doing all those things. What was the composition of the stones? That's why I'm here." She repeated that statement multiple times.
>
> Dr. Jeffries said, "It often takes six to eight weeks, and they send them to Texas, so I can't answer that question right now." The patient left the office while Dr. Jeffries said, "If we can be of any further service just contact us." Dr. Jeffries then went over to Carmen and said, "May I ask where the stone analysis was?"
>
> Carmen said, "It will take me ten minutes to get into the old chart."
>
> Dr. Jeffries told her, "Ten minutes is all you get." He then mumbled under his breath. "She [the patient] was pissed off, she waited that long, and she's being passive aggressive."

Dr. Jeffries, similar to all the doctors I observed, always tried extremely hard to meet the patients' needs. In this case, there was no diagnosis, and both the doctor and the patient were dissatisfied. By this time, I had realized that each of the medical assistants takes primary responsibility and has a one-on-one working relationship with one of the doctors. Carmen was a close working partner for Dr. Jeffries.

Not only did the medical assistants assist in retrieving data required for a diagnosis narrative, they also assisted in generating such data. For this task, they often interacted with multiple different bureaucratic and social institutions:

> Marsha then embarked on an extended task of trying to get prior authorization for a CT scan for the next day. It was with [a patient's insurance company]. She said, "I am calling for Dr. Patel," using his name. Next, she was placed on hold for an extended time before being transferred to someone else. When she didn't get the satisfaction of obtaining an authorization number, she hung up the phone and said to herself and to the phone that was hung up, "You can't even help me." She then made another phone call. Given the chance to talk with a customer service representative from the insurance company, Marsha said, "I was put on hold forever. I never heard of that number. Dr. Patel's NPI

number[6] is 5845669328." She had a habit of asking for the person's name that she was speaking to and kept notes in her stenographer's pad. On the computer screen in front of her there was a scanned image of the [medical insurance] card displayed larger than actual size, approximately 7" x 11" [instead of 3 1/4 x 2 1/4]. She was reading the numbers from it. This became an extended episode of not only talking about a prior authorization for a CT scan but also for bone scan. Once she was on hold so long she simply hung up. She made a comment about trying to do this now because she knew that she would be too busy for the rest the afternoon. Marsha was talking to someone and said, "Hopefully, I'm not calling them back. I wrote her name down and I just want to double-check with you [that the authorization number was valid]. The other person I talked to didn't seem very helpful. It's crunch time. The surgery scheduling at Maplewood Hospital won't let them do it without prior authorization. This is for a prostate biopsy." All types of clinical information was requested and Marsha said, "The patient had a PSA, then a biopsy, and the biopsy was positive for cancer, so there were no symptoms." The person she was talking to kept asking for symptoms and Marsha kept saying, "There are no symptoms." Marsha then had to provide more information about the biopsy that had been performed on October 25. Marsha conversed with two or three different people; she kept writing their names down on the stenographer's pad. When she finally did get the authorization number, she said, "Can I repeat that number for you? I just want to know your name." She then had to call surgical scheduling and convey the authorization number to prepare for the surgery the next day. After she hung up, she realized she had been on the phone for approximate 35 minutes trying to get this preauthorization. Marsha indicated that that was usual. She concluded by saying, "Their attitude makes me mad and then it's my 'snitty' attitude myself which I don't like."

I understood that what I was seeing was the work of assembling vast amounts of data (narrative elements) used to proceed with the cultural practices at my field site. Eventually, I came to understand that the diagnosis itself was a causal sequence and that pronouncing the diagnosis was the work of the doctor. I gained an appreciation for how important the computers were to do this work. They were important because the narrative elements that were combined by causal sequences and narrative schemas had to first be acquired before the "diagnosis story" could be told in a convincing way. I realized that the only socially authorized individuals to tell diagnosis stories were doctors, a key finding of the entire cultural practice of an outpatient medical office visit. The medical assistants were the support people, providing information to the doctors and implementing requests from the doctors. As mentioned, most of the time and most of the effort of the office personnel in this setting was devoted to this process. The next excerpt is specific to the software used for the electronic health record.

Dr. Stein went over to Carmen and said, "Do I have to send her a task[7] or can I tell you?"
Carmen asked, "What do you want?"
"I want to get a CT scan of the chest. Put on the requisition 'renal mass, rule out metastases.' I prefer that he have it done at Maplewood so I can look at the film myself."
"I'll take care of it for him [the patient]." In this way, Carmen circumvented the computer software and simply focused on getting the job done.

Although the Electronic Health (Medical) Record contained data and narrative elements necessary to function, it never made a diagnosis – only doctors can do that. The electronic medical record has become such an integral part of providing care that Marsha used the initialism EMR as a verb. Marcia was putting a patient in the room and she gave the patient a very cheery greeting. She was all smiles and in an extremely good mood. She was working with Dr. Stein and turned to him and asked, "Dr. Stein, do you want me to set up the procedure room or do you want me to EMR the patient in Room Two?"

Gathering diagnostic narrative elements requires teamwork

On another occasion, there was a computer malfunction, and Dr. Jeffries asked Carmen about the next patient. Carmen was able to give a detailed medical history using medical terminology, correctly sequenced, and summarized the patient's history of the present illness. She knew the names, doses, and frequency of the patient's medication as well as his urinary volumes from when the patient had a Foley catheter placed in the emergency department of the hospital.[8] Observing this interaction, I had the distinct sense that she was performing better than most resident physicians did. Most importantly, Dr. Jeffries trusted the information and was able to complete the office visit.

This level of detail was not a unique experience. The next day, Dr. Jeffries said, "Carmen, how is Mr. Schmidt doing today?" Again, Carmen provided a complete medical history. This type of accuracy and reliability was a result of Carmen reading each consultation and reviewing the medical records before scanning them into the electronic chart. On one occasion, Carmen was eating lunch and opening mail. One of the pieces of mail was a three-page consultation letter from someone at the state university. Carmen read the report carefully and thoroughly before filing it.

The previous section documented the amount of work it took to assemble a complete set of data to provide patient care, but these observations made me realize the amount of personal responsibility the medical assistants took to involve themselves in this process. Not only did they know what information was needed to provide patient care, but they also understood the content and were able to provide it when the doctor requested it.

On one occasion, Dr. Jeffries stepped out of an exam room to ask Carmen, "What dose does Toviaz come in?"[9]

Carmen said, "4 mg and 8 mg but she is already taking 8 mg."

On another occasion, Dr. Jeffries started asking a question but Carmen stopped him mid-question and said, "It's printing out the stuff right now."

Dr. Jeffries asked, "Carmen, how do I manage signing all these attestations? I end up doing it all twice." He was referring to how the electronic medical record forced redundancy in order to clear out his inbox.

Carmen said, "I'll do it. Just go see the next patient." She did his repetitive computer work so he could see another patient.

On another occasion, Dr. Jeffries asked Carmen, "What are these [papers]?"

Carmen replied, "I'll figure it out. Just sign them."

Again, she was doing the tedious paperwork so he could do the work appropriate to his level of training.

The medical assistants also worked as a team and cross-covered for each other effortlessly, frequently asking, "You need anything?"

Carmen said to Marsha, "I have to send that out for cytology."

Marsha said, "Okay."

Carmen responded, "You're the best."

Later, Carmen asked Barb, "Hey Barb, can you print me an insurance paper?"

Barb replied, "It's on the counter," indicating that she had anticipated Carmen's need and supplied the insurance information before Carmen actually asked for it.

Marsha had to "unlock" one of the electronic medical records and asked Carmen for help. Carmen said, "I'll do it for you because I love you."

Marsha replied, "You're the best."

Carmen followed that with, "You always help me when I'm in a jam."

After a busy day, Barb said, "We survived it."

Marsha said, "We are good at what we do. We run like a well-oiled machine."

Indeed, the office did "run like a well-oiled machine." These people truly have affection for one another. I use these observations to support my impression that the *doctor* is actually a group of people working in a highly coordinated fashion toward a unified goal: patient care. Consider the following description of teamwork to obtain diagnostic narrative information.

This vignette demonstrates other types of "narrative components" for a diagnosis-narrative. Carmen and Dr. Jeffries are in direct contact with each other while performing a prostate biopsy, positioning the ultrasound machine to achieve a critical diagnostic narrative component – the biopsy report.

If a patient was to have a biopsy during clinic hours, Carmen and Dr. Jeffries could complete an entire biopsy routine wordlessly. Each anticipated the movements of the other and they coordinated the many different sequences flawlessly and efficiently. Carmen and Dr. Jeffries worked silently, not even looking in the same direction at the same time, but each completing what the other was doing. Dr. Jeffries would point to the ultrasound screen, and Carmen would move the rollerball, making exact measurements of the size of the prostate. During the punch biopsy, the tissue specimens were collected and labeled efficiently.[10] Both gave instructions to the patient at different times without any duplication of effort. Consider the following action:

Carmen said to Dr. Jeffries, "Your biopsy is ready."

"I'll be right there." Dr. Jeffries was sitting at the computer documenting his second-to-last patient of the day. He sat there typing with his index fingers. I noticed that he typically uses the computer farthest to the left at the doctors' charting station with high stools and countertop. Carmen went to give the patient the informed consent.[11]

He continued typing. Eventually Dr. Jeffries said, "Are you ready, Carmen?" Shortly thereafter, Dr. Jeffries got out of the chair/stool, and they both went into the procedure room. Dr. Jeffries told the patient, "Just sit back and let us drive the machine. We're ready to roll." He spent a significant amount of time positioning the patient, "Sit on the edge and then lie down. . . . Roll on your left side. . . . Scoot your hips to the edge of the table . . . Move your shoulders here, and then roll your shoulders towards the opposite end over there." This took a lot of verbal direction and working with the patient. Dr. Jeffries then sat on a stool next to the ultrasound machine, which was on his left. The patient was on his right. Carmen had a procedure setup table covered with a blue drape over the top. They both had blue gloves on. She took the drape off, revealing six small bottles filled with fluid. There was also a trigger-activated biopsy gun with an incredibly long needle, approximately 8 to 10 inches. Carmen stood behind Dr. Jeffries, and Dr. Jeffries spent half the time looking at the ultrasound machine screen and half the time looking at the patient. Dr. Jeffries warned the patient that there can be a pressure sensation and told him to "Breathe out." The ultrasound probe had a portal to insert the trigger-activated biopsy needle. The probe was plastic, approximately fourteen inches long, including the grip handle. Dr. Jeffries inserted it and the patient expressed some discomfort with mumbled utterances but no verbalizations. Dr. Jeffries said, "Dr. Stein said he doesn't like this one. It can't scan."

"Why can't it read?" Carmen wondered aloud. "I'm not going to question things."

Carmen and Dr. Jeffries were working silently but in a highly coordinated way. At times Dr. Jeffries would point to the ultrasound screen. Carmen would move the rollerball and pushed the button in different areas and different times. Dr. Jeffries said, "Here you can see the seminal vesicles. That's prostate tissue. The bladder is quite empty, which is good." He then said to the patient, "I would like to rotate the probe," and made a comment that he didn't like this [referring to the position] . . . "It's hard to [insert the syringe and/or loaded punch biopsy syringe]."

As Dr. Jeffries rotated the ultrasound probe intra-rectally, the patient had a grimace on his face.

Dr. Jeffries said, "This is not hurting me a bit. [Pause] Is it hurting you?"

As Dr. Jeffries was pointing to the screen and Carmen was pushing the button. She said, "Apex, right?" There was again more nonverbal communication.

After taking measurements, [dimensions of the right and left lobe], Dr. Jeffries said, "There is going to be some poking and some stinging," then inserted a syringe with very long needle through the sheath and injected clear fluid. The patient winced with discomfort. He did it twice more, removed the syringe, and inserted the next instrument. It was a hollow tube with a hollow needle, cocked like a gun. It made a loud click as Dr. Jeffries pushed the button. When it was inserted and the trigger was pulled, I could see the needle stab into the prostate on the ultrasound machine displaying live video, demonstrating the hollow core needle penetrating through the prostate. During the process, Dr. Jeffries explained they were going to take 12 of those core biopsies, six on each side. Throughout the procedure, the patient essentially had his eyes closed.

After that phase of the procedure, Dr. Jeffries asked the patient, "Do you have children?"

"A son, and my daughter is a nurse. How many more?" He repeated this exact same question again having not gotten a response the first time.

After the patient asked the second time, Dr. Jeffries replied, "Does it hurt?"

The patient asked [for the third time] "How many more?"

"Two. It's normal to have blood in the urine and blood in the poop." Dr. Jeffries turned his attention from the patient back to the ultrasound machine saying, "We never printed the dimensions."

Carmen replied, "Yes. I'm on the ball." After that, Dr. Jeffries removed the probe. It was covered in blood.

After completing the procedure, Dr. Jeffries told Carmen that the ultrasound images with the measurements needed to be scanned into the medical record. Overall, it was an impressive demonstration of teamwork.

Three weeks later, the patient and his wife returned to get the results of the biopsy. Before we entered the exam room, the two of them were speaking in a foreign language. Her English was much better than his. When Dr. Jeffries entered the room, she immediately asked, "What was the result of the biopsy?"

"There's some good news and some bad news. I brought this copy of the report for you to keep." He then went over the results, explaining that there was some "pre-cancer," continuing, "The bad news is the cells were abnormal, and it would require a repeat prostate biopsy to know for sure. The good news was there was no definitive prostate cancer." After he explained this to the patient and the wife, Dr. Jeffries asked, "Is that something you'd be willing to do?"

Without asking her husband, she replied, "Of course. We want to know the answer. We want to catch it in time."

Dr. Jeffries replied, "Yep." They went on to schedule it on October 5. Dr. Jeffries left the room and typed detailed notes in the computer.

The wife's comment, "We want to catch it time," will be discussed later in Part 4. This vignette again illustrates the dichotomy of experiences between the doctor and the patient during gathering of narrative elements. This is best illustrated by the statement, "This is not hurting me a bit. [Pause]. Is it hurting you?" Although I will highlight the importance of shared experience later, this type of dichotomy of experience is a source of criticism that doctors are insensitive or inattentive to patient concerns. Despite this seeming divergence of experience, the need to "catch it early" creates the motivation to continue the process until the patient experience merges with the doctor's experience.

Clinical time and narrative time

The compression of time into a clinical encounter by retrieving past narrative elements or components, procuring future narrative elements, and assembling stored data related to a schema for a diagnosis narrative describes the work of the medical office. The element of time is fundamental to narrative – it is what relates episode one to episode two. In order for the doctor to create a diagnostic narrative, he has to fill in the blanks of the diagnostic narrative schema. Even if it required multiple office visits, the definitive diagnosis narrative was never complete until all of the diagnosis elements were procured. It is in this way that I view the social practices described in this section. As my research progressed, I realized that assembling diagnostic narratives is only one part of a larger healing ritual experience, as I mentioned earlier. However, it is one of the more important activities. As I continued my research, I discovered yet another critically important component of the diagnosis narrative. There was something more than words or stories residing in the computers, something I discuss in the next chapter.

To conclude this section about assembling narrative elements for a diagnosis narrative, I provide one more vignette demonstrating the complexity of working with multiple computers simultaneously and sorting through multiple access points into various computer systems simultaneously in the context of completing a single clinical encounter. I am still attempting to portray how doctors practicing Western biomedicine achieve a diagnosis.

> Dr. Stein came out of the exam room and began documentation at the podium with the barstool-type chairs. He was actually using three separate computers and looking at paper reports simultaneously. On the left-hand computer, he was looking up lab test results in one software program on the right-hand computer he was documenting an electronic health record associated with the University. He was also incorporating data from the paper reports. The middle desktop computer he used to log onto Maplewood system to look at diagnostic images. Periodically through the session, he was checking his email on his laptop. Dr. Stein was creating his documentation in the same electronic health record used by the others. I did notice that he was the first physician to use all ten fingers to type (The others used different versions of hunt and peck.). Interestingly enough, he would open the same templates but only filled them in partially and then went to the preview of the consultation letter and edited heavily in the actual letter as opposed to entering the data in the database format of the electronic health record. He was meticulously writing a narratively structured document instead of a computer generated amalgam. He asked Marsha, "Could you call a telephone number?"
>
> Marsha scribbled the telephone number on a paper towel and said, "I need patient information to do that." Dr. Stein gave her the billing sheet that had the patient's demographic information printed on it and then Marsha called to get the results of the scrotal ultrasound. She later reported to Dr. Stein, "Dr. Moss did the ultrasound himself and there is no report, but there were some labs."

After Dr. Stein finished his consultation letter in the electronic health record, he took the papers to the large square Formica box with the slit for disposing of protected health information and discarded the papers. I personally have seen them in four different offices and they are emptied by a standardized shredding service. There is a life cycle of paper in this office. Whenever paper documents are received, they are scanned into the electronic medical record. As the medical assistants prepare the patients for the office visit, they print the relevant scanned images of previous paper records so that they are available to the doctor. As indicated, when the doctor has incorporated whatever he deems relevant into the note and is finished with the paper documents, they are shredded.

Embedded in this vignette is a clue to one of the key findings of this research. Included in the process of assembling data, Dr. Stein has one of his computers open to the Maplewood server where he can view the CT scan directly himself instead of relying on a printed report of the CT scan from a

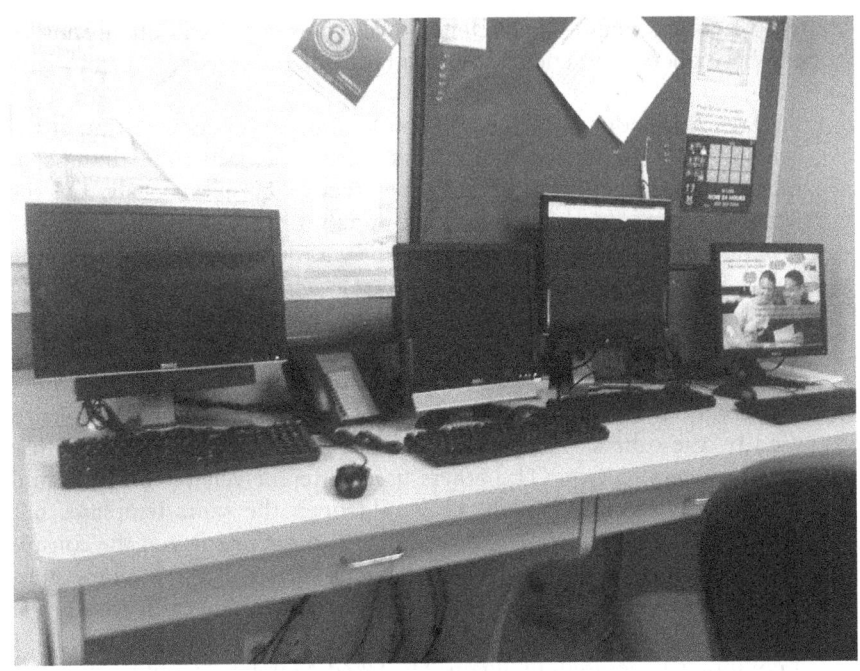

Figure 4.1 Computer screens at the doctor's workspace

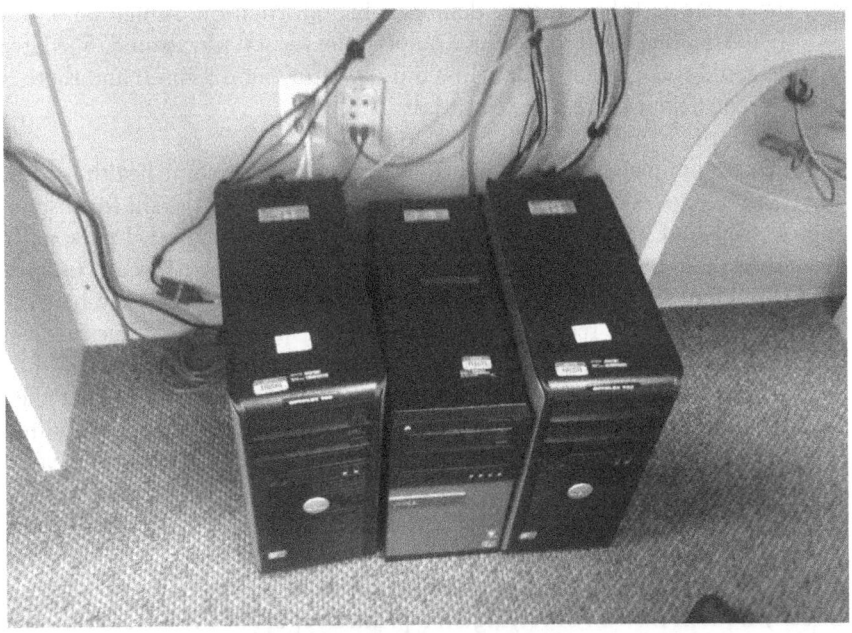

Figure 4.2 CPU towers for the doctor's workspace

radiologist. In the next chapter, I emphasize the relative importance of this type of data compared to all other types of data.

Notes

1 A stent is a wire mesh that keeps a tubular anatomical structure open.
2 Dr. Williamson was a resident physician, still in the early phase of his training.
3 The lowest number indicates no symptoms.
4 Medial sulcus is a slight depression between two lobes of the prostate gland.
5 Here, Dr. Stein is trying to trap Dr. Williamson into self-incrimination because those are not the anchor descriptors of the Likert scale on the AUASS.
6 NPI number, or National Provider Identifier, is a standard unique identifier for healthcare providers. It is a way to track physician activity. It was mandated by the Health Insurance Portability and Accountability Act of 1996 (HIPAA).
7 A "task" is similar to an email, but one that is embedded in the electronic medical record. It is a way for different members of the "distributed cognitive network" to communicate with each other, but it also creates an audit trail, recording who knew what when, and who was assigned responsibility to obtain the data or narrative elements.
8 This type of phrasing is typical in a medical environment, often filled with euphemisms – for example, "placing" a Foley catheter is uncomfortable for the patient.
9 A medication for benign prostatic hypertrophy (BPH) that helps increase urine flow.
10 A punch biopsy uses a hollow needle which is thrust into the organ to yield a core of tissue that is removed for microscopic examination.
11 Informed consent refers to a signed document that signifies the patient understands the procedure and accepts the risks of the procedure.

References

D'Andrade, Roy. 1995. *The Development of Cognitive Anthropology*. New York: Cambridge University Press.

Foucault, Michel. 1973 [1994]. *The Birth of the Clinic: An Archeology of Medical Perception*. New York: Vintage Books.

Frank, Arthur W. 1995. *The Wounded Storyteller: Body, Illness, and Ethics*. Chicago: University of Chicago Press.

Hutchins, Edwin. 1995. *Cognition in the Wild*. Cambridge, MA: MIT Press.

Mattingly, Cheryl. 1998. *Healing Dramas and Clinical Plots: The Narrative Structure of Experience*. Cambridge: Cambridge University Press.

Tomasello, Michael. 1999. *The Cultural Origins of Human Cognition*. Cambridge, MA: Harvard University Press.

5   Spatial cognitions

Michael Tomasello characterized our sensory-motor world in terms of spatial relations. He states:

> All mammals live in basically the same sensory-motor world of permanent objects arrayed in a representational space; primates, including humans, have no special skills in this regard. Moreover, many mammalian species and basically all primates cognitively represent the categorical and quantitative relations among objects as well. These cognitive skills are evidenced by their ability to do such things as:
>
> - Remember "what" is "where" in their local environments, e.g., which fruits are in which trees (at what times);
> - Take novel detours and shortcuts in navigating through space;
> - Follow the visible and invisible movements of objects (i.e., pass rigorously controlled Piagetian object permanence tests – some stage 6;
> - Categorize objects on the basis of perceptual similarities;
> - Understand and thus match small numerosities of objects;
> - Use insight in problem-solving.
>
> (Tomasello 1999: 16)

Nick Enfield pointed out that hand motions can symbolize genealogical representations and that these symbolic spatial relationships are maintained over time (Enfield 2005). The ability to maintain spatial relationships over time is a key cognitive skill that I will richly describe with the following data.

As I mentioned earlier, the medical assistants and doctors assembled the information required to conduct an office consultation prior to the doctor walking in to greet the patient. In this section, I want to focus on a very specific but vitally important subset of that process: reviewing the imaging tests. The following vignette demonstrates the importance of viewing images to the work of the doctor. Similar to other types of narrative elements, the doctors and those that worked with them were frustrated if they were unable to assemble all the necessary narrative elements. Dr. Stein demonstrates how vital it is to review radiologic images. Another clue to the importance of these spatial cognitions is the amount of time as a percentage of all activities that occurred in the office – approximately 50 percent, dramatically more than the time spent with the patient. I came to realize these spatial cognitions were narrative elements that they were actually more essential for this office than verbal or numerical narrative elements.

Dr. Stein then resumed clinical work by reviewing a CT scan image. He addressed the medical student: "The CT is easiest for me because I have more familiarity with it." He did look at the cyst on the kidney and said, "That looks benign.[1,2] It is eccentropic[3] on the left." As he was changing the slices on the CT image using the rollerball on the mouse, he pointed to and touched the screen. He would repetitively use the rollerball to "flip through images," similar to animation images, outlining the top and bottom of the cyst, saying, "That is the kidney. There is a stone . . . another stone." He then commented, "This is so slow." As he was continuing to review the CT scan he said, "This is so small." Dr. Stein finalized his review of the CT scan by saying, "I don't think it's worth an operation for that little thing." He then walked around the corner into the administrator's office. Coming back with administrator and pointing to the computer, he said, "There's the hourglass of death." He was referring to the time it took to download the image. He asked the administrator, "What has been done about it?"

She said, "I contacted the people at the hospital. I asked the director and they told me the only other option was to drop a cable to improve data transfer [from the hospital across the street]."

Dr. Stein said, "How do we know they're doing anything about it?"

The administrator replied, "We purchased new computers. You approved the expense. It's not the computer. It's the data transfer that is preventing more rapid opening of the images."

At that point, Dr. Stein repeated himself, "How do we know it hasn't just been dropped and forgotten about?"

The administrator replied, "It's been on our list. The only thing we can do is keep reminding them that we want something done. They work on their own time schedule and are not responsive to what we were hoping for. It will continue to be slow until they drop the new cable."

Dr. Stein replied, "You have not calmed me down."

The administrator replied, "Apparently that's not something I can do."

After the exchange with the administrator, Dr. Stein came back to the computer and, looking at the computer with a medical student, said, "So I would not operate. I don't even want to try the MRI because it's going to drive me nuts."[4]

The doctors flipped through the images while gazing at the screen. This activity was intense work. As the ethnographer, I watched hundreds of hours of this activity. Through conversation concurrent with the activity, I learned that the doctor formed a three-dimensional cognition with this process. The heated anatomical discussions associated with this practice revealed that the doctor was adding another layer of detail every time he flipped through the images. This vignette is important because it highlights Dr. Stein's dependence on reviewing the data-dense images and the frustration of data transfer that delays his work. Dr. Stein made a decision ("I don't think it's worth an operation for that little thing") simply by reviewing the CT scan image. The diagnostic narrative components were all contained in the reconstructed three-dimensional image. This is in contrast with the work involved in acquiring the other aspects of the diagnostic narrative mentioned in the previous section. The relationship between the two activities is that all the office work leading up to obtaining this CT image preceded Dr. Stein reviewing this CT image. Similarly, recall how hard Marsha worked with the insurance company to get a pre-authorization to perform a diagnostic imaging test. In most cases, imaging exams were key diagnostic narrative components:

Dr. Stein asked Dr. Jeffries to look at images on the computer screen, saying, "There was a CT scan in 2007, 2009, and 2011." He had all three scans open on computer screens simultaneously. Dr. Stein said, "This area was present in 2007 and 2009, but looks cystic and non-worrisome. But on this 2011 scan it looks markedly different," as he was scrolling through sequential slices of the CT images of the mass.
Dr. Jeffries said, "Sounds like you need to do a biopsy, or surgery."
A few minutes later, Dr. Jeffries came walking down the hall and said, "What did you decide to do?"
Dr. Stein replied, "Get more information with an ultrasound."

Although Dr. Stein said this with an absolute deadpan voice, never taking his eyes off the computer screen, it is vital to understand that this response was complete sarcasm: he said the exact opposite of what he meant to say. An ultrasound would provide no additional helpful information. After consulting with his most trusted colleague and staring at the images repeatedly, he needed to make a decision; he needed to make a diagnosis.

I will return to this case in the next section, but at this point is vital to understand the role of three-dimensional cognition as part of the diagnosis narrative within a healing ritual. Indeed, I will present several other identical cases and relate how the doctors deployed the images in the ongoing ritual. It is only important to note that this was a daily activity, not something rare. As I continued fieldwork, this same issue – personally reviewing images – was consistently present in every setting and by all doctors. The next vignette combines the concept of the three-dimensional cognition and the computer as repository of the diagnostic narrative components of images. The setting is the university cancer center, where urological cancers were discussed by oncologists, radiation oncologists, urologists, and internists. As described in the methods section, I followed Drs. Stein and Jeffries to this Wednesday morning conference where I met other doctors in this multidisciplinary practice group.

> A multidisciplinary care conference (MCC) is a type of tumor board where doctors from multiple disciplines review difficult diagnoses. The presenter solicits multiple opinions about diagnosis and management. At one session, a radiologist was reviewing images. He said, "This case shows a very large tumor on the kidney. I'm going to show the coronal images,[5] just to get a different vantage point. With the MRI of the abdomen, we can see the renal vein [pointing, speaking, and flipping through the MRI slices simultaneously]. We can track this all the way back. This is the renal vein and it is normal, not affected by tumor."
>
> Another case at MCC, the presenter was demonstrating the effect of chemotherapy by comparing two images simultaneously, "This mass is almost the size of the entire liver and after chemotherapy, it shrank to this – the size of a marble. But as we move down here [using the roller-ball on the mouse], you can see that the bladder wall is still thickened [indicating the source of the primary tumor]."
>
> Dr. Stein presented a case at MCC, and toward the end he showed a PET[6] scan of the patient. This is different because it was in color, not in the black, white, and grey of the CT scan or MRI. The PET scan displayed coronal images, and Dr. Stein scrolled through the images toward the front and back through different slices. He said, "Try to get a sense of the size and shape of the tumor." As he was doing this, the computer screen was freezing, causing a delay in the presentation of the images, fragmenting the three-dimensional perspective. The computer's central processing unit froze and an error message came up on the screen that indicated there wasn't enough memory. This was followed by another error message that read "low memory detected." Part of the problem was that he had left all the previous scans opened, but minimized – there were four or five of them. When the computer froze again, Dr. Stein stopped, saying, "I just wanted to show that PET-CT scan because it's so clear."

I will return to the three-dimensionality of cognitive processes as I present more data, but at this point, I was convinced that the diagnosis was something the doctor arrived at by reconstructing not only the physiology (laboratory tests) but also the anatomy and pathology, using the various imaging techniques. My overwhelming impression at this point as an anthropologist was that I was observing the new and improved version of what Michel Foucault called "the clinical gaze" (Foucault 1973, 1994). I also recognized that my earlier observations of collecting diagnostic information to fill in the diagnostic schema during the office visit included collecting not only laboratory values such as PSA, stone analysis, urine analysis, but also the CT, MRI, and other films for the doctor to review. Sometimes they were stored in the computer system downtown, sometimes they were stored in the computer system at Maplewood, and sometimes patients brought them in on a CD.[7] This chapter discusses how there is another "storage area," inside the doctor's mental life.

The practice of using the computer mouse and the rollerball on the mouse to flip through slices of the CT or MRI was ubiquitous. Every urologist did it during every clinic session. Other specialists, the oncologist and the radiation therapist, also practiced the same visualization technique. Using the human cognitive abilities to maintain abstract spatial relationships and manipulate them, these doctors were creating cognitive holograms by flipping back and forth through two-dimensional images – essentially converting them mentally into three-dimensional cognitions that could cognitively viewed from multiple perspectives. The reason they repeatedly flipped back and forth is that their attention was directed toward a particular anatomical structure, determining where it began and ended. The next pass through the CT file would add other anatomical structures to the cognitive hologram they were creating mentally. Later ethnographic data reveals how these surgeons draw upon these mental holograms during surgery. As technology changes, perhaps the computing systems will create the holograms automatically on a more routine basis. Currently, 3-dimensional renderings are used selectively. But at this time, the finding that "spatial cognitions" are important to clinical practice is an important part of this research.

The following is an observation during oncology inpatient rounds at the university. Dr. Spangler is an oncologist (a subspecialty of internal medicine dealing with cancer care – in this case urologic cancers). She works closely with Dr. Jeffries and Dr. Stein.

The resident was presenting a follow-up case, and Dr. Spangler asked, "What about the EGD [esophagogastroduodenoscopy]?"[8]
The resident said, "You want to look at the pictures?" He got the chart off the rack and showed Dr. Spangler the printed digital images that were taken during the EGD.
Dr. Spangler said, "That is nasty and makes me want to puke."
The resident said, "There were three liters of fluid that were taken out."
As Dr. Spangler was looking at the printed digital picture she said, "Oh, my God! Oh, my God, that is disgusting!" One of the residents commented, "It's odd that a doctor is making a statement like that."
Dr. Spangler said, "No, we're sympathizing with her [the patient]. She wants to know where the necrosis in the stomach was, where the obstruction was. Oh, crap."

The resident said, "We should strongly consider hospice."

Dr. Spangler came back asking, "Where's the pressure causing the necrosis coming from? Look at the last [CT] scan. Anatomically I can't see it." The stomach was necrotic,[9] even though it was pancreatic cancer. "There must be some compression, potentially of an artery or vascular structure causing the necrosis in the stomach," Dr. Spangler continued, "She's a walking skeleton." At that point, everyone stopped what they were doing and Dr. Atlas, a fellow,[10] pulled up the image of the CT scan and scrolled through the slices demonstrating the tumor, scrolling up and down until they could anatomically connect the pancreatic cancer to the area of the stomach that was black on the printed digital images from the EGD.[11]

Oncologists typically reviewed films during the multidisciplinary conferences in conjunction with urologists, radiation oncologist, and radiologists. I later learned that Dr. Spangler reviewed each image personally outside of actual clinic time. She also reviewed on an as-needed basis, as in the preceding example. The radiologist's report, of course, required the radiologist to perform the same cognitive reconstruction of a three-dimensional image by reviewing different planes (cross-sectional, sagittal, and coronal) and flip through the sliced images to mentally create the holographic image. This is based on the mammalian and primate cognitive abilities described by Tomasello and described earlier in this chapter. The natural extension and progress in technology is to allow the computer to construct the hologram. I met Dr. Rivers at the Multidisciplinary Care Conference where he interacted with Dr. Spangler, Dr. Jeffries, and Dr. Stein. I followed him to his outpatient office. This next vignette occurred demonstrates the cognitive processes and software necessary to create such a hologram:

Dr. Rivers (a radiation oncologist) started explaining the entire process to me. He said, "I use the CT scan in the room next door and that is aided by MRI if necessary. It's my job to outline the prostate and specifically the contour of the prostate. I'm also responsible for indicating the area in which the radiation field can occur." He used a computer system with software very similar to commercially available Adobe Photoshop, outlining the anatomical structures on the CT image itself. "Here I'm outlining the lymphatic bed. It's my job to actually read the film and identify the structures. When I'm done, I turn it over to the person who works on designing the angles and the dose. There is anywhere from two to five different angles. The object is to maximize the dose on the organ that needs to be treated. There are official standards of tolerances for dose irradiation for non-affected organs and this view represents those numbers in a dose volume histogram. The CT images of specific organs are reconstructed on the computer."

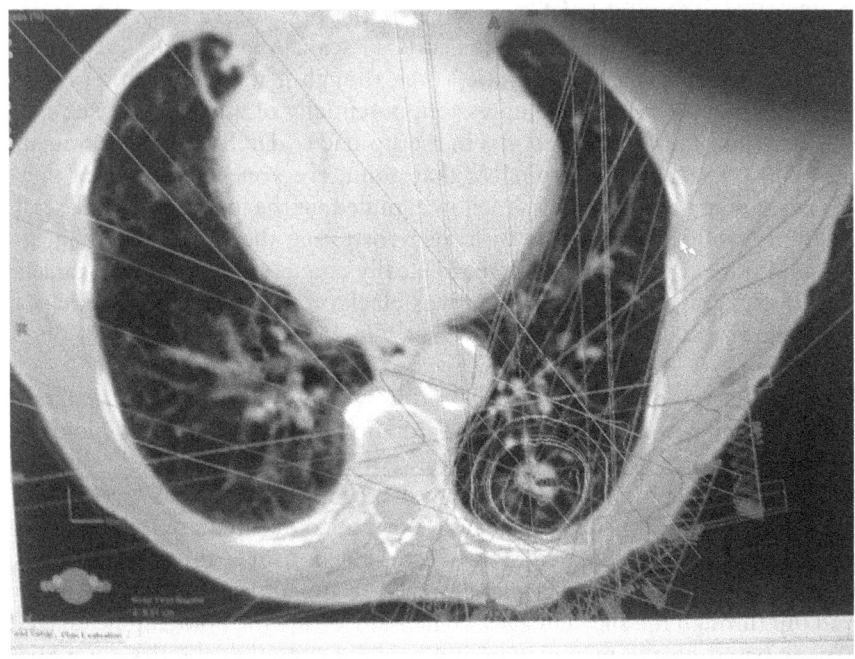

Figure 5.1 Anatomical structures outlined on CT with dosimeter plan overlay

Dr. Rivers is using the computer and the CT scan image in the same manner as Dr. Jeffries and Dr. Stein, identifying pathologic organs and outlining them anatomically. Again, this diagnosis is for treatment planning. The treatment planner cannot make the diagnosis; his job is merely to calculate angles and radiation doses to fit into the standardized tolerances. Because the connection of diagnosis to therapy is so closely linked, it is difficult to isolate them. I will explore therapy later. For now, I want to demonstrate how all physicians use the rollerball on the mouse while interacting with computer images and to illustrate the next logical formulation in current medical practice, the hologram.

Dr. Rivers was speaking aloud, presumably telling me what he was doing, never taking his eyes off of the computer screen. He was looking at the CT scan, using the rollerball on the mouse coming back and forth using slices to re-create and identify structures in the same way that I saw Dr. Stein and Dr. Jeffries do hundreds of times. He said, "In radiation oncology we use stereotactic body radiation therapy. We are able to use a 4D CT, meaning the CT scan monitors the maximal excursion of the organ being treated during respiration. That way we can limit the

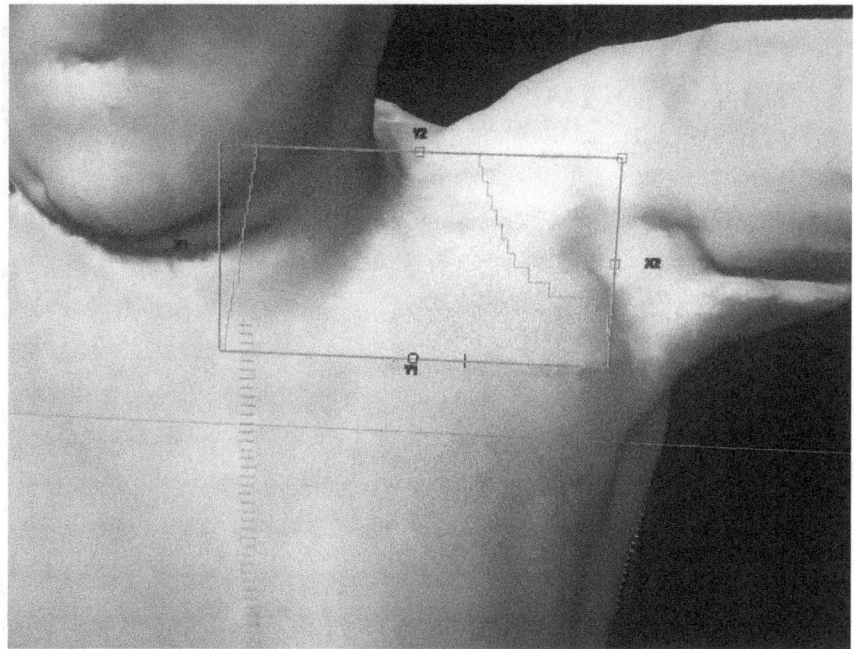

Figure 5.2 Computer-generated hologram composite from CT images

amount of radiation to that tightly defined boundary. The only other alternative is to extend the boundary to make sure we treat the entire diseased organ."

The radiation oncology treatment center had computing power far in excess of the computers that Drs. Jeffries and Stein used in their outpatient office. Five computer towers filled a small room. These computers connected all the CT scanners, MRI, the treatment planning computers and the CyberKnife machine. They were able to create actual holographic avatars. In other settings, the doctors used human cognition.

Many anthropologists describe spatial cognitions (Danziger 1998; Kirill and Dwyer 2009; Levinson 1996; Levinson 1998). Many cognitive scientists from other disciplines describe similar cognitions. They describe "the body" in relationship to *exterior space*. The cognitions I was observing showed the doctors reconstructing and maintaining mental images from each slice of the CT or MRI and re-assembling them into a three-dimensional object related to spatial cognitions with an emphasis on the *interiority* of the body. I do not know of other ethnographic data describing

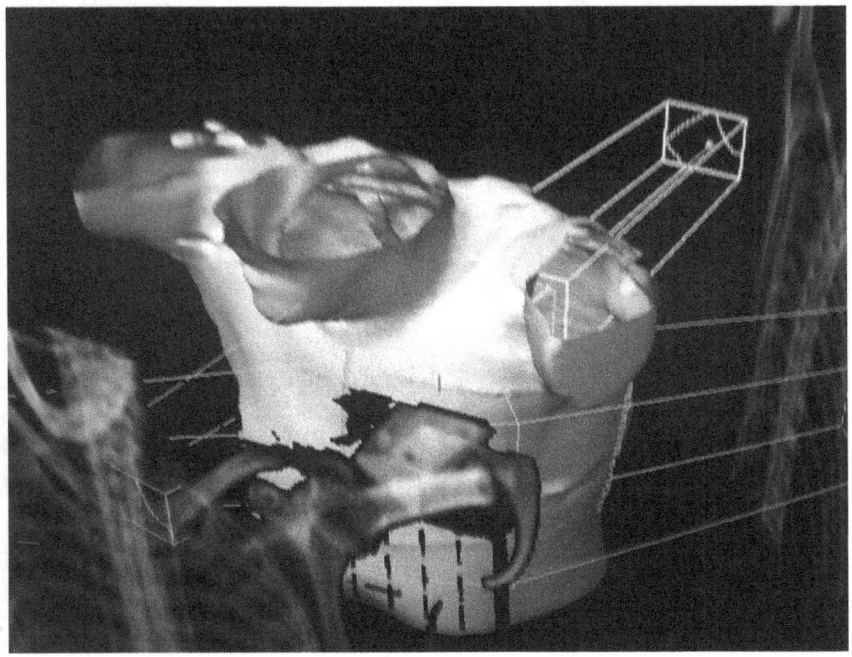

Figure 5.3 Hologram with cutout treatment plan

such interiority of space within the body, yet when I describe surgery, the interiority of the body (surgical operation) had occurred originally within the mind of the doctor embedded in a diagnostic narrative.

Notes

1 A cyst is a mass that is filled with fluid as opposed to solid; the significance is that cysts are very rarely malignant.
2 Benign means not malignant – cancer is only one type of malignancy.
3 This word means that the mass is growing outward from the contour of the kidney.
4 There is a much higher data load burden for an MRI compared to a CT scan.
5 Coronal, the last of the three axes to create the three-dimensionality, slices the images of the body starting at the belly button and proceeds toward the spine.
6 PET scan, or positron emission tomography. This image is generated by a radio-nuclide (radioactive) particle injected as part of glucose (sugar). The images demonstrate physiology instead of anatomy.
7 CD is an acronym for compact disc, a mobile storage form for imaging data.
8 A combination of a fiber-optic light and tube to directly visualize the esophagus, stomach, and first part of the small intestine.
9 Necrotic refers to dead tissue.
10 A fellow is a doctor that has finished post-graduate training during residency and continues further training in an even more specialized discipline of medicine. In

this case, Dr. Atlas was board certified in internal medicine and his fellowship was in oncology.

11 EGD is an acronym for esophagogastroduodenoscopy, a direct visualization of the esophagus, stomach, and the beginning of the small intestine.

References

Danziger, Eve. 1998. Introduction: Language, Space, and Culture. *Ethos* 26(1):3–6.

Enfield, N. J. 2005. The Body as a Cognitive Artifact in Kinship Representations: Hand Gesture Diagrams by Speakers of Lao. *Current Anthropology* 46(1):51–81.

Foucault, Michel. 1973 [1994]. *The Birth of the Clinic: An Archeology of Medical Perception.* New York: Vintage Books.

Kirill, V. Istomin, and Mark J. Dwyer. 2009. Finding the Way: A Critical Discussion of Anthropological Theories of Human Spatial Orientation With Reference to Reindeer Herders of Northeastern Europe and Western Siberia. *Current Anthropology* 50(1):29–49.

Levinson, Stephen C. 1996. Language and Space. *Annual Review of Anthropology* 25:353–382.

———. 1998. Studying Spatial Conceptualization Across Cultures: Anthropology and Cognitive Science. *Ethos* 26(1):7–24.

Tomasello, Michael. 1999. *The Cultural Origins of Human Cognition.* Cambridge, MA: Harvard University Press.

6   The doctor tells the
diagnostic story to the patient

As mentioned earlier, every office visit began by collecting all the relevant clinical information and reviewing the imaging studies. So far, the doctor formulated the "diagnosis narrative," but I have not described how the narrative is told, spoken, and to whom. Contrary to "healing" as a function of the patient telling the narrative, I saw the doctor speaking and telling the narrative to the patient. After the preparation of gathering the narrative elements and formulating a diagnosis narrative, the doctor went into the room prepared to convey that narrative he made prior to ever greeting the patient. Consider the following examples:

Dr. Jeffries explained to me, "The next patient has a seven-millimeter renal mass and it doesn't meet criteria for biopsy. The patient is complicated because she's on warfarin."[1] He went into the room, which was the first time he ever met the patient, and the patient was sitting there with who appeared to be her mother. He opened by saying, "I know you know why you're here. I'm just going to say it anyway. There's a lesion on your kidney or a mass or tumor. Those words are all bad because they have negative connotations. What you really have is just a small bump on your kidney. I can't promise you that it's not a malignancy, but by imaging criteria and size criterion I'm not thinking of doing surgery. I'm sure you have a lot of anxiety and your doctor has a lot of anxiety."

The patient said, "That's true."

Dr. Jeffries resumed, "I have a suggestion that may resolve all the problems. I recommend a biopsy with the interventional radiologist at Connaught Cancer Institute. They will not only evaluate the seven-millimeter lesion to determine whether it needs to be biopsied and if necessary also do a biopsy of the kidney for the nephrologist because she is considering lupus nephritis."[2]

Dr. Jeffries left the room first and I stayed behind, and then the mom and the patient started laughing aloud. While laughing, the patient smacked the mom on the back with a magazine and said, "I told you there's nothing to worry about." As they were leaving, the patient said, "Goodbye. Thank you."

This was a very short visit with a new patient. The patient was pleased simply to hear good news, that she did not have cancer. There was no long explanation; the patient and the patient's mother simply accepted the diagnosis (not cancer) at face value. I witnessed this same social dynamic many times. I had now figured out the story (diagnostic narrative), the storyteller (the doctor), and the audience (the patient). The perlocutionary power of the diagnostic story (diagnostic narrative) is powerful. The important thing is that the doctor always made the decision about what the story was going to be about before seeing the patient. In the next vignette, Dr. Stein introduces himself and discursively steers the patient to his pre-formulated diagnosis:

Dr. Stein was also seeing a patient in consultation, so he approached the patient as if he never saw him before. He reviewed all of the medical records prior to entering the room. Upon entering the room, he said to the patient, "I reviewed all of your scans before coming in, and I think I know why you're here, but I'd like to have you tell me why you think you're here."

"I've had many biopsies – at least eight or nine – because my PSA is 19."

Then Dr. Stein told the patient, "My partner sent you to me for a different type of biopsy."

"Is it going to hurt?"

Dr. Stein said, "We're going to do it in the operating room and so they will give you something so it won't hurt, but you won't be totally asleep." He took a plastic model of a prostate off the windowsill and said, "This is the direction the needle usually goes to do a prostate biopsy, but Dr. Patel wants a different type of biopsy so we can check a different part of the prostate. The needles will go through the skin. They go in at a different angle," and then using his index finger demonstrated the direction and area of the prostate he was going to biopsy. "Everybody is worried about a cancer that hasn't been diagnosed. It's mysterious why your PSA is high, because your prostate is not that big." Dr. Stein leaned back and said to the patient, "So do you want to do this biopsy?"

"Yes." At that point, the patient went out to the appointment counter.

Dr. Stein said to Barbara, "Schedule him for a saturation prostate biopsy and if they ask, they can set up the operating room similar to brachytherapy."[3]

Again, there was a diagnostic story: "I've reviewed all your scans before coming in." He already has in mind what he is willing to offer the patient. The patient can accept or decline, but the diagnosis does not change. Even when patients think they know the story and convey clinical data, it is the prior review of the diagnostic narrative schema, including review of the images by the doctor that is used for the diagnosis narrative. The following vignette demonstrates this point:

Dr. Stein was looking at the CT scan and again said, "There it is. I can't memorize T1, T2, but blood is white," pointing to the screen and then said, "No, I'm sorry. That's the gallbladder. These images are loaded backwards. They are labeled 'R' on the left side of the screen which is standard, but as I take progressive slices lower, the liver becomes more prominent on the right side of the screen." He pointed out that discrepancy to the medical student. After standing in the hallway reviewing all the images, Dr. Stein went in to talk to the patient. He sat down on the stool looked straight at her and said an introductory hello.

The patient said, "Let me help you out. I had proteinuria,[4] so I was sent to a nephrologist[5] initially, had an ultrasound and the CT scan, and then the MRI. I saw Dr. Patel who asked for the second opinion by you."

Dr. Stein allowed the patient to complete the entire chronology and only then said, "We just spent 20 minutes reviewing the different scans. I think the probability is that the cyst is benign. It's a very low probability that it's cancer." While Dr. Stein was in the room, he only made direct eye contact with the patient. "I recommend you come back in six months to have a checkup with the CT scan."

We left the room, and as the patient was leaving the room passing the podium she said, "Thanks for the reassurance."

Similar to the preceding example, most patients do not challenge the diagnosis or management. The following example was one of the few exceptions I observed. In this example, the patient's challenge did not change the diagnosis or the recommended management:

Dr. Stein said to the medical student, "I'm done [with patients] but I have a CT scan of a patient I saw last week here on this CD." He then inserted the CD into one of the computers at which point he turned to the fourth-year student saying, "This one loads quickly because all the data is on the CD and we don't have to wait for data transfer." Dr. Stein then went over with the medical student a detailed analysis of the CT scan saying, "The tumor is in the top location."

Dr. Jeffries was finishing his clinic session and said, "Is that for a partial?"

Dr. Stein said, "I haven't done an open partial in the longest time but this would be a crazy partial. This was an incidental finding. After I looked at it, there are difficulties in doing this laparoscopically.[6] It's behind, not anteriorly. It's too big. Eventually I need to call the patient and tell him 'I think you need surgery.'"

Dr. Stein then called the patient on the phone, saying, "I got your discs. This is a sizable tumor. My preferred approach is to do an open surgery. . . . I agree with you but it's not in a good position. It's too big to attempt it laparoscopically. I am doing a lot of surgery laparoscopically, but in my judgment this one would be too difficult." He then used his index fingers to count space on the countertop before saying to the patient, "It's about 6 to 7 inches in diameter. . . . I'm looking at the CT scan while I'm talking to you. . . . You would be laying on your side. . . .

The incision would be under the ribs. We could use stitches or staples whatever you prefer. . . . We can put stitches in if you would like." There was a short pause and then Dr. Stein said to the patient on the phone, "I'm trying to do as many cases laparoscopically as I can, but this one is in the wrong place, is too big, and the tumor itself will be difficult to resect.[7] . . . You're also going to need a CT of the chest to make sure it hasn't spread. A lot of urologists would simply do the easier surgery which is the total nephrectomy but it's always better to do a partial nephrectomy, even if you can't do it laparoscopically. I'm pretty aggressive laparoscopically and I have a lot of confidence. . . . I don't want to do this one laparoscopically. I don't know what [another surgeon] would do." After getting off the phone, he turned to Dr. Jeffries, saying, "It's oblong, exophytic as well as endophytic, deep in the retro peritoneum," and then asked Dr. Jeffries, who overheard the entire conversation with the patient, for a second opinion.[8]

Here, I want to point out that like every diagnosis, the culmination of gathering narrative diagnosis elements results in the review of the three-dimensional mental image of the cancer in relationship to location in the body, surgical access points, and technical considerations in acting on the diagnosis. When Dr. Stein pronounced this more complex diagnosis, he refused to change his opinion, despite multiple challenges from the patient. Dr. Stein dismissed newer and more sophisticated technology based on the three-dimensionality of his diagnosis. He also defended his diagnosis against the cultural model of newer technology always being better.[9]

Diagnostic storytelling

The concept that the doctor makes the diagnosis and tells that story to the patient without benefit of input from the patient seems harsh, yet it was a consistent finding throughout the research. I provide one more example of telling the story of a diagnosis. This time it occurred on the inpatient oncology service:

The resident was presenting another patient who had metastatic prostate cancer. "He is a patient of Dr. V. He is on a Phase I drug versus placebo trial[10] and scheduled to receive radiation therapy but was admitted with nausea and vomiting. They gave him the Zofran this morning.[11] Apparently, the patient also tripped and fell."
Dr. Spangler summarized the management by saying, "Get physical therapy and occupational therapy on board."
A resident was reading one of the reports and the report had a big word in it. He said, "I'm not even sure what that means. The previous CT scan was done in January."
Dr. Spangler replied, "That's probably just fatty liver."

The oncology fellow then turned to check the labs on the computer, "The PSA was 260." He showed a graph of the PSA, and although it looked like a stock market graph, the end of it went straight up.

Dr. Spangler asked, "What was the calcium level? So why is he puking?"

One of the residents guessed, "Hepatitis?"

Dr. Spangler asked, "How much narcotics is he getting today? We still haven't solved the issue of why he's puking."

"Could it be the radiation . . . or brain mets?"[12]

Dr. Spangler said, "I'll be a monkey's uncle if it's brain mets." She thought about it, "I guess I can't be an uncle but I'll be a monkey and aunt," then used it as a contraction, "a *m'aunt*." She was referring to the fact that prostate cancer rarely metastasizes to the brain, unlike lung cancer in a previous patient. "We need to talk to him about goals. We're pretty much done. We need to send him back to his primary care physician. He is living off half of a lung. He needs to finish out the course of radiation therapy, get occupational therapy and physical therapy." She then pulled out her iPhone to look at the calendar, calculate how much longer the radiation therapy would continue, and made the statement, "He has two or three weeks more to go [with radiation therapy]. We've maxed out what we can. . . . It's a hard discussion. Social work needs to find out what he needs at home. This is going to be a hard discussion, because he just lost his daughter and his mom. He's dying and is only 55 years old."

The diagnosis was "He's dying." Dr. Spangler reached this conclusion while sitting around a table in the hospital reviewing CT scan reports, the medical record, laboratory data, and other diagnostic narrative material. It was not an inconsequential diagnosis. Compare this "story" to the story earlier that concluded "It's probably not cancer."

I started fieldwork naively looking for illness narratives and now I have described diagnosis narratives. Earlier, I suggested the two were complementary. Consider briefly the absurdity of patients telling their own diagnosis narratives. Could a patient tell a story with enough cultural authority to schedule an operating room in a hospital and hire a surgeon to do whatever surgery the patient demands? Conversely, the diagnostic story can eventually become incorporated into an illness narrative, but I was exploring diagnosis narratives at this point in my fieldwork. It was clear what a heavy burden these stories carried for the doctors – there is little room for error because of the profound impact the stories had on the life of others.

Many patients require a combination of treatment modalities, so doctors from different disciplines discuss cases at multidisciplinary care conferences (MCC) once a week. Multidisciplinary care conference is a social space where doctors debate alternative treatment plans. Although doctors pronounce the diagnosis with certainty with patients, they share the ambiguity, the uncertainty, and the conflicting demands of difficult cases at MCC. In addition to coordinating care, this venue is a place where doctors can share their uncertainty, the uncertainty that is never part of the diagnosis story shared with the patient:

Multidisciplinary Care Conference was held at the main Connaught building at the university, and, as the name implies, physicians from different
disciplines discuss cases and solicit input from others. The auditorium
seats about a hundred people. The room is, oddly enough, shaped like
a kidney, with curving, convex outer walls and drooping ceiling, with
a feeling of theater in the semi-round, focused on the screen where CT
and MRI images are displayed.

At about seven o'clock, there was a rush of people into the room, and Dr. V
(an oncologist) started presenting a case. She gave a very short presentation that had the following structure: (1) chief complaint, (2) diagnosis
of bladder cancer, (3) CT showed lymph nodes, (4) biopsy and biopsy
results, (5) chemotherapy summary.[13] It was an extremely abbreviated
clinical presentation, and then she presented the following, "The patient
has reached the limits of chemotherapy and I'm presenting her to see if
there is something else that can be offered." The resident slowly scrolled
downward, through multiple image slices, to the bladder, showing a
thickened bladder wall.

At that point, Dr. Stein spoke and said, "That's all? No lung mass?"

Dr. V said, "I'm conflicted. I can't imagine putting her through surgery given
the fact that she's had liver mets."

Dr. Wright (a resident physician) said, "She's only 40 years old."

Dr. V continued, "At a minimum she can get cryo[14] to the bladder, and
someone can look in the bladder."

Dr. Rivers, the radiation oncologist, added, "I don't think surgery is
warranted."

Dr. Stein said, "The patient has liver mets and the bladder looks terrible, but
she's not about to die from her cancer. Just do a quick cystectomy. The
literature supports surgery."

Dr. V seemed surprised and with an upward tonal inflection of her voice
asked, "She's not [about to die from her cancer]?"

Dr. Stein said, "The cystectomy could be considered palliative with potential
for survival benefit."

At that point, Dr. Rivers said, "There isn't any support for that in the
literature." His statement sparked a very robust discussion among
multiple participants. The urology residents participated freely despite
their junior status amongst a mixed group of faculty physicians with
residents.

They reviewed the CT scan again and Dr. Stein said, "We do lots of things
we don't have Level I evidence in the literature."[15]

Dr. Rivers said, "I don't think that's reasonable."

Dr. V asked, "Can you cryo the lymph nodes?"

Dr. Rivers said, "Not this one. It's too close to the femoral nerve," and pointed directly to the CT scan on the screen.

Dr. V said, "So you're both willing to offer cystectomy with an informed discussion?"

Dr. Stein said, "Are you going to talk to the patient with a frown on your face?"

Dr. V replied, "I think it's crazy . . . they [other cancer centers] could call us crazy."

"I completely disagree with that statement," responded Dr. Stein.

Dr. Wright said, "She's got one met and she's young and healthy."

Dr. Stein continued, "I don't agree with what you said."

Dr. V responded, "If you can find a couple of experts to say that, it's going to need a lot of informed discussion."

Dr. Stein then said, "Maybe the discussion should be with someone who does surgery."

Dr. V said, "You'll get your chance."

The conversation then drifted to the quality of life and Dr. Stein said, "When the patient leaves the hospital, she will be on an oral diet, have an ileal loop, and within six weeks will be back to a normal lifestyle."[16]

Dr. Rivers said, "What happens while she's off chemotherapies for six weeks for surgery? Don't you risk rapid recurrence of her disease?"

Dr. V and Dr. Stein continued presenting opposing viewpoints. Dr. V said, "The time issue is important. We have to present it as if we don't know if it's going to blow up with metastatic disease. There is other disease there. We're just not seeing it. I can talk to the patient whether or not she should have surgery, but with metastatic disease, her long-term chances of survival are 5 percent. This would be a big lifestyle change."

"Where'd you get this 5 percent?"

"Clinical reports and patient studies."

"Is she like those other patients in the study?"

"Do you want to see her first so I don't pollute her mind?"

Dr. Stephens (a junior faculty urological surgeon) said, "I can see her later today and review it with her."

This is a somewhat unusual case, illustrating the edge between the known and the unknown. The fact that the medical opinions are so disparate is important. Also, note the "consent" comments. There is very little confidence in a consensus of what the patient will be "consenting" to undergo. This vignette highlights the importance of telling the interim diagnosis story correctly, but the case is notable because the doctors are having difficulty recommending a treatment because they cannot persuade even themselves of what the correct story should be.

Although they are comfortable sharing disparate opinions in this setting, by the time the doctor talks to the patient, the "story" has already been determined, even if it required the input from colleagues such as in this case.

Continuing the rhetorical re-formulation of prostate cancer management, one need only consider the tongue-in-cheek conclusion to the following case.

Dr. V presented the second case. "This case is a patient with a PSA greater than 10, Gleason score 3+3, stage II.[17] The patient didn't want treatment but was offered hormonal treatment. He then went to the Voter Hospital and heard about 'seeds'[18] but eventually chose no treatment. When he was reevaluated for his cancer at the Voter Hospital, they repeated the biopsy and it showed no cancer. So this patient actually went from biopsy proven disease, an interlude where he declined treatment, followed by a biopsy that was negative for cancer, and he never received treatment from 1997 until now. Throughout that entire time, he refused to have a PSA, but he's being presented at tumor board because his primary care physician did a PSA by mistake and the PSA turned out to be 250. The patient has arthritis and the Voter Hospital did a bone scan, which couldn't exclude mets. The patient had some obstructive symptoms, controlled with Flomax."[19] The assistant for the presentation was scrolling throughout the bone scan, again using the roller on the mouse.

No one responded throughout this entire time until Dr. Stein said, "You can use finasteride[20] to improve voiding symptoms. You can say he made the right decision at the time." The group then discussed what the standard of care was in 1997. Dr. Stein continued, "The patient had peri-neural invasion with prostate cancer, and the second biopsy that was negative was false assurance that the cancer was gone; this patient's been living with his cancer for the entire time."

Dr. V said, "There are multiple cores."

Dr. Stein said, "He put himself on watchful waiting 15 years ago, and this is just his 15-year follow-up."

At that point Dr. Rivers said, "It depends what you presented to him, a smile or frown." [This sarcastic comment referred to the previous case when Dr. Rivers and Dr. Stein disagreed and Dr. Stein said, "Are you going to talk to the patient with a frown on your face?"]

The doctor offered this patient treatment and the patient declined. Dr. Stein totally reframed the case from one of non-compliance to "He put himself on watchful waiting 15 years ago, and this is just his 15-year follow-up."[21] Using his deadpan humor, Dr. Stein presents the paradox of the treatment not directly related to the diagnosis and an implied re-evaluation of how to present the diagnosis to the patient. Dr. Rivers quickly reiterated the moral dilemma, saying, "It depends on what you present to him, a smile or frown."

Here in the arena of uncertainty of the MCC, doctors are re-evaluating the moral dimensions of pronouncing a diagnosis.

Notes

1 Warfarin is an anticoagulant drug, so any biopsy or surgery would have increased risk.
2 Lupus nephritis is a form of chronic kidney disease secondary to an underlying disease (lupus). It is important here because to remove part of the kidney would only further decrease kidney function.
3 Brachytherapy is the placement of small "seeds" into the prostate that emit high-dose, localized radiation therapy as a treatment for prostate cancer.
4 A word that means protein in the urine – normally there is not supposed to be any detected, but if it is, it is considered abnormal.
5 A nephrologist deals with medical problems of the kidney.
6 Laparoscopically means surgery done through a metal tube the diameter of about a finger – all the cutting, clamping, and visualization instruments are inserted through this tube inserted into a one-inch incision. Other instruments are sometimes also inserted through other small incisions simultaneously.
7 Resect means to cut out of the body.
8 Exophytic means growing outward; endophytic means growing inward.
9 Personal communication from Jerome Hoffman, MD, Professor Emeritus UCLA, who likes to use this phrase when discussing overdiagnosis.
10 Phase 1 trial is the first time a new pharmaceutical or chemotherapeutic agent is used in humans. The research is designed only to determine if it is safe. There is no intent to even determine if it is useful or not. It is like experimenting on human guinea pigs.
11 Zofran is a drug used to treat vomiting, especially in patients receiving chemotherapy.
12 Met or mets is shortened slang for metastasis, or spread of the cancer to distant organs.
13 There is a rigid organizational schema for case presentations common to any clinical setting, typically called a "history and physical," although it is used in many settings. Dr. Jeffries usually always provided me with such a summary when I was seeing patients with him.
14 "Cryo" is short for cryotherapy, a type of tissue destruction caused by extreme cold temperatures.
15 There are multiple grading systems in evidence-based medicine to describe the quality and believability of the research.
16 Ileal loop is a surgery where the bladder is removed and part of the small bowel is brought to the abdominal wall for use in draining urine out of the body and into a bag.
17 The Gleason grade tells you how fast the cancer might spread. It grades tumors on a scale of 1–5. You may have different grades of cancer in one biopsy sample. The two main grades are added together. This gives you the Gleason score. The higher your Gleason score, the more likely the cancer is to have spread past the prostate: Scores 2–5: Low-grade prostate cancer; Scores 6–7: Intermediate (or in the middle) grade cancer. Most prostate cancers fall into this group; Scores 8–10: High-grade cancer. www.ncbi.nlm.nih.gov/pubmedhealth/PMH0001418/
18 "Seeds" refers to radioactive pellets inserted into the prostate gland tissue as a form of treatment.
19 Trade name for tamsulosin, a drug that relaxes muscles near the bottom of the bladder, making it easier to get urine out.

20 A drug that inhibits an enzyme that changes testosterone into a more potent form of testosterone; this means that it is an anti-androgen, or male hormone medication.

21 Watchful waiting is allowing the patient to avoid treatment for prostate cancer and only treat if he becomes symptomatic. This is to be contrasted with active surveillance, where the goal is to time the surgery correctly, minimizing the horrific complications while still getting maximal therapeutic benefit.

7 Joint attention to the diagnostic narrative

Joint attention to a spatial cognition-diagnosis narrative

It was common, but not universally practiced, to re-demonstrate the CT scan review with the patient as a method of explaining the diagnosis. Consider the next observation.

> Dr. Stein was talking to the medical student at the documentation counter-top, pointing to a CT scan, saying, "Look at that renal mass."[1] He was flipping through the CT scan slices as I had seen him do innumerable times. He said, "This is the nephrogram phase and this is the collecting system phase.[2] You check the non-contrast images to check for kidney stones," and then he motioned Dr. Jeffries to join them, "Look at this scan." Dr. Jeffries, Dr. Stein, and the medical student were all staring at the CT scan. I naturally drifted over to view the scan as well. All four of us wound up staring at the CT scan. Dr. Stein said, "Here's the kidney." He used his finger to point to the image of the kidney on the CT scan as he reviewed the various slices of the CT image from the top to the bottom and back, finding the optimum slice to demonstrate what he wanted to demonstrate to the rest of us. Finding the optimum slice, he used the arrow location on the screen, controlled by the mouse, making circular motions with the arrow to point out the abnormality on the kidney that was suggestive of a renal mass. Dr. Stein said to Dr. Jeffries, "This would be difficult to do robotically." Dr. Stein then scrolled through the slices incessantly and when I looked over to see what he was doing, I saw him reviewing the sagittal[3] slices of the CT scan instead of the cross-sectional images.[4] Dr. Jeffries and I saw another patient and when we came out of the room from that office visit, Dr. Stein was still looking at the exact same films of the patient with the renal mass. Dr. Stein said to Dr. Jeffries, "Take a look at this. Do you agree this is a stone?"
> "Yes."
> "They completely missed it when they read this CT." Dr. Stein then asked the patient to come out from the exam room and brought them over the

computer and pointed to the kidney stone on the CT scan and said to
the patient, "This is where the kidney stone is, right between the bladder and prostate."
The patient asked, "Is my prostate large?"
Dr. Stein said, "Yes, and I'm surprised you're not having symptoms."
Dr. Stein asked Dr. Jeffries, "Will you do the ureteroscope and take care
of the stone, and I'll take care of the renal mass later? I'm going to get
a CT-guided biopsy of the renal mass." They agreed to schedule it at
Maplewood. All these scans were on a CD that Dr. Stein had put in his
computer. Dr. Stein said, "Maybe the patient should keep the disc."
Dr. Jeffries said, "I wish we had a way to upload those images to our
computer."
Dr. Stein then put the CD in an envelope and told the patient, "You need to
bring the disc to the operating room so that they could look at it when
you get there."

There are three levels of persuasion in this vignette. First, Dr. Stein persuades himself that he has made the correct diagnosis; then he persuades Dr.
Jeffries his own diagnosis is more correct than the one in the written report
by the radiologist; and finally he brings the patient out of the exam room
and points out exactly where on the image demonstrates his rationale for
treatment. Narratives persuade. In this case, he suggests treatments, one by
Dr. Jeffries for the kidney stone and the definitive cancer treatment subsequently scheduled with him.

Again, a similar observation demonstrates the same format:

Dr. Jeffries walked down the hallway to an exam room, saying to the people
in the room, "I want to show you on x-ray – would it be possible for
you guys to come down here?" referring to the documentation desk
with the computers to view the CT scan images. There was an older
woman who didn't speak English, a younger woman who translated
from Spanish, and a five-year-old little boy who was running up and
down the hallway. Dr. Jeffries said, "This is the CD [with the CT scan
on it] you brought me." Then standing in front of the computer screen
he turned around and faced the patient and the interpreter.[5] He did a
demonstration on his own body saying, "This is like a special telescope,
so this is the right side and you're looking in this way." He then turned
back to the computer and used the computer mouse rollerball, scrolling through the CT slices, saying, "We're moving inward here from the
belly button."
The younger woman was translating everything he said. At one point, she
said, "Can you put them back side-by-side?" She was referring to the
two kidneys. Dr. Jeffries adjusted the slice image on the CT scan and
there was a prolonged time of interpretation directed at the patient by

the interpreter. The interpreter was pointing at the computer screen, comparing the normal kidney to the one with the abnormal mass. Then the patient asked about the pain in the leg.

Dr. Jeffries said, "I can't explain the pain in the leg. Perhaps the tumor is growing inside the blood vessel, and it's partially obstructed, and that's giving you discomfort in the legs. In order to find that out I want to get an MRI," saying each letter of MRI very slowly with long pauses in between, "to make sure there isn't any blockage. This needs surgery as soon as possible. I'm going to have Carmen [the medical assistant] arrange the MRI."

The issue of insurance coverage came up. By this time, Dr. Jeffries was standing behind the appointment counter and said, "Tell her you don't have to worry about that." He then interacted with Carmen and asked, "Should I talk to an administrator?" He decided that that he would take care of it. He repeated his admonition, "You don't need to worry about that. We're from University Medical School." The interpreter asked about the pain and Dr. Jeffries recommended Tylenol. He specifically said, "She can't take aspirin or Motrin or anything else like that because it will interfere with her ability to have surgery. Put your feet up on the pillow when you get home from work and take Tylenol."

These types of interactions demonstrate joint attention: the doctor and the patient are both attending to the CT image. There is verbal dialogue and visual input that results in a shared cognition, that cancer is the diagnosis. It seems that the side-by-side comparison of the normal kidney with the diseased kidney was essential to understanding as the patient asked to have that image re-demonstrated. This allowed a comparison: there is a general conception that the right side of our bodies should be similar to the left, if inverted. The important part of this vignette is that with a language barrier, the "language" used is allowing patients to see the three-dimensional images for themselves. In this example, as well as the previous one, note that three or four people were all sharing joint attention to the CT scan image while discussing the diagnosis. The same was true at MCC. Many people can simultaneously share the joint attention described by Tomasello.

The next vignette was introduced earlier, demonstrating that the diagnosis was a three-dimensional cognition of the doctor. Here, I extend the vignette to demonstrate the next step in the healing ritual, persuading the patient of the diagnosis.

Dr. Stein asked Dr. Jeffries to look at images on the computer screen, saying, "There was a CT scan in 2007, 2009, and 2011." He had all three scans open simultaneously. Dr. Stein said, "This area was present in 2007 and 2009 but looks cystic and non-worrisome. But on this 2011 scan it looks markedly different," as he was scrolling through the mass with the rollerball of the mouse.

Dr. Jeffries said, "Sounds like you need to do a biopsy, or surgery." A few minutes later, Dr. Jeffries came walking down the hall and said, "What did you decide to do?"

Dr. Stein replied, "Get more information with an ultrasound."

Quite a bit later Dr. Stein brought an elderly gentleman and two other people, one male, one female, out to the same computer screen and showed them the images. He then said, "The problem is they log you out. It's torture getting logged out. I'm trying to see patients, and it continually logs me out." He then asked them to step back in the exam room to see if they could use the computer there. Approximate five minutes later he had re-opened all the images again on the computer screen. Bringing them back to the computers, he informed them, "The first CT scan was in 2007, the second one was 2009, and this is the CT scan in 2011. It looks a little more solid. I've been studying all of these [referring to the images], and on MRI things look slightly different. This [pointing to the image on the screen] is what I'm worried about. We can do a needle biopsy into this area. The surgery would be coming in like this [indicating on his own body the direction of the incision and how to reach the mass demonstrated on the CT image]."

"What if it's cancer?" the patient wondered out loud.

"I would only take this part of the kidney out. You only have one kidney. I would not take the whole kidney out. You think about it and let me know what you want to do."

The patient replied, "I'll think about it."

Dr. Stein then said, "I apologize for the very long visit. This was very complicated and difficult to figure it out." At that point, the family group left the office.

Again, there are multiple levels of persuasion. When making a major diagnosis, Dr. Stein asks Dr. Jeffries to confirm his three-dimensional interpretation of the CT scan image. Here the argument includes a change over four years. Instead of left should be similar to right, the argument is that there should be constancy over time; change is a marker for growing cancer. Dr. Stein is again quite careful, and, instead of merely relying on a verbal description, he shows the images to the patient to persuade them of the cancer diagnosis. In many other examples, he simply uses the rhetorical argument, "I've reviewed your CT scan images carefully," before ever attempting to pronounce a diagnosis to a patient.

These examples show how the doctors use visual images to explain their recommendations for treatment to patients. Again, in an attempt to "see" what is really going on at the field site, I explored and confirmed the diagnosis is three-dimensional, a cognitive hologram constructed cognitively that replicates diseased anatomical structures. The spatial cognition that makes up part of the diagnosis narrative describes the interiority of the body – the story of the body, reminding me of the trope of the body-self-story. These examples also demonstrate one form of "rhetorical persuasion," sharing the image with the patient, using joint attention to achieve agreement to the diagnosis narrative.

The next vignette occurred in an inpatient setting. The urologist could not take the computer into the patient's room, so he printed an image from the CT scan and took it with him to pronounce the diagnosis.

> Immediately after he came out of the room, I went in to see the patient and she said, "Here is the kidney cancer. He told me that, based on the size, he would be able to take all of it out and I will be cured. See, here is the cancer [the patient points to the CT image]."

Diagnostic storytelling and the ratchet effect

Cheryl Mattingly describes something similar to a diagnostic narrative using examples from when she worked at the World Bank in Calcutta.

> I recognized that stories were not just told after experience but were constructed while people were still very much in the midst of action. This active storytelling played a critical role in team strategizing about

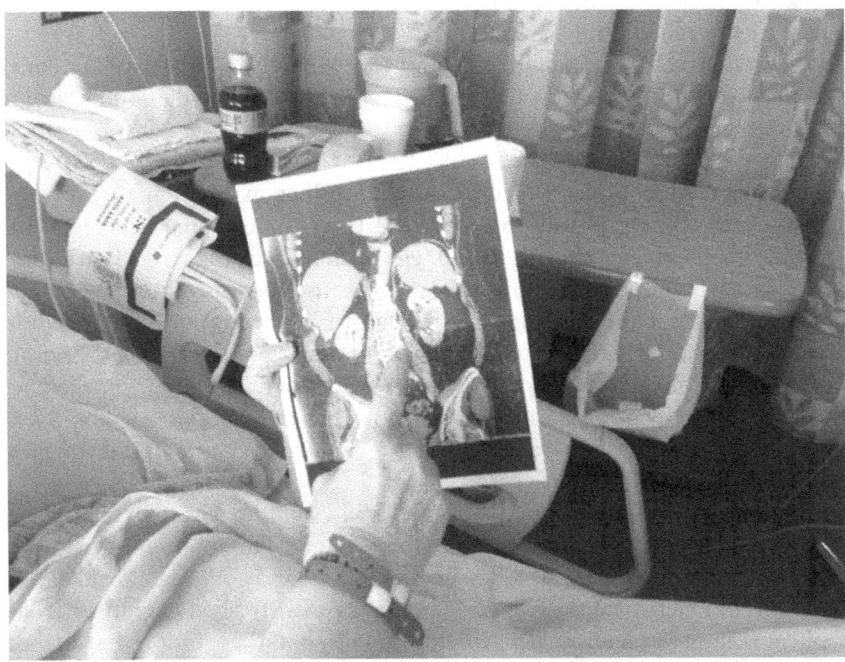

Figure 7.1 Patient using a CT image to explain the diagnosis to the researcher

how to turn project implementation in more desirable directions. Thus I began to examine narrative as an aesthetic form with rhetorical powers, on which could become a persuasive tool for convincing others to see the world in a certain way.

(Mattingly 1998: 5)

In a similar way, diagnostic stories have rhetorical power, convincing patients to engage in therapeutic actions.

Patients are socialized to live within the world of the medical diagnosis

The patient has to be convinced the diagnosis is correct and agree to the treatment. Recall Jerome Bruner describing Emmy's ability to accept or reject the experience of the "other." When the doctor and patient use joint attention to the same diagnostic narrative, patients begin to use medical jargon and present themselves – their illness story – using the diagnosis narrative as an important part of the story. This was a rather consistent finding. My data demonstrate that, in the setting of the clinical encounter, patients acknowledge the audience (doctors and nurses) and contribute to a shared narrative using the lexicon of biomedicine. At this point, there is a shared culture as the doctor and the patient speak the same language. Consider the following examples.

Dr. Atlas [an oncology fellow working with Dr. Spangler] had seen the second opinion patient from Benedict Hospital and when he came back to the charting room, he presented the case to Dr. Spangler. "This the 57-year-old man with a family history of prostate cancer in both the uncle and questionably the father. Diagnosis was made in 2008, PSA was 6.5. Ultrasound guided biopsy showed Gleason eight, high-grade lesion, PSA at that time was 10. After surgery the PSA was undetectable and then became 0.3, 0.4 which was a rise and at that time patient was put on Lupron[6] in March of 2009. It was stopped approximately year ago and last month PSA rose to 0.3 with the increase in the back pain. The patient sought second opinion."

Dr. Spangler pointed out that the only imaging that was done was five years ago. "They needed a bone scan." She then explicitly told Dr. Atlas, "What patients need from a second opinion: number one, they need to know whether something's been done right or wrong in the previous care the patient received, and, number two, they need to know what to do next." She then specifically went over the details of the case with Dr. Atlas and pointed to the pathology report, saying, "It's right there – two positive lymph nodes – which means that it was locally metastatic at the time of surgery. One could argue that he should have been treated with androgen deprivation therapy right at that time," and referred to a journal article in *New England Journal of Medicine*. "We are going to have to couch that very gently if we tell him about it. She talked about whether the patient should have had radiation oncology treatment at that time. "Does it change things in the big picture? No, not really. The guy's on hormones and he should stay on hormones. There's been no imaging and it's been four years later. He still can be considered castrate because it takes a long time for the testosterone level to rise and she said if you do reimage, there's a good chance you might find something.

Dr. Spangler went into the room with Dr. Atlas to talk with the patient. Dr. Spangler asked him, "Since this is a second opinion, it is very important for me to know what you are expecting."

The patient said, "They weren't aggressive enough. They haven't done any scan since my diagnosis." The patient talked about getting the robotic prostatectomy and then being put on Lupron. He said, "I'm having back pain and that worries me. I use the word worried; I could use the word concerned." He then pointed to a lump in the back. The patient described his case with a lot of technical jargon. When Dr. Atlas initially talked to him, the patient said, "My PSA was drawn on a regular basis and it was seven after surgery. It was undetectable after that." He listed the specific dates that the PSA was undetectable and said, "I'm fighting it." Dr. Atlas was looking for the most recent PSA which he didn't have. The patient said, "I'm sure it is in the folder [the folder the patient brought with him]." He went through the papers, found the lab letter with the result on it and gave it to Dr. Atlas.

Dr. Atlas examined this lump on the back and he said, "It is a lipoma – a fat tumor under the skin."

Again, the patient used all medical jargon. He used words like "undetectable," "radical prostatectomy," "Lupron," he knew the date of every specific PSA level and the PSA value result. He presented the data in chronological order. He knew every scan that he had and the result of the scan. In summary, he actually told Dr. Spangler, "I know this is stage IV . . . I just decided I should find out if we should be doing something else."

Dr. Spangler asked, "What was your previous response to Lupron?"

"Shortness of breath."

"That isn't a known side effect of the medication."

"I had to go to the emergency room twice. It was a very stressful time . . . we had to move in with my son."

Dr. Spangler informed him, "You need to go back on the hormones. You need a complete evaluation, including a CT scan of the thorax, a CT scan of the abdomen, a CT scan of the pelvis, a bone scan and a dexa scan for bone density. We need to check for pathologic fractures from osteoporosis – a side effect of prolonged hormonal therapy." After Dr. Spangler told him of the extensive workup, she turned to Dr. Atlas and added blood tests to his workup. "Are you going to follow up here at Connaught?"

The wife asked, "Are all the scans going to be done at Connaught?"

"Yes, Connaught has its own CT scan and its own MRI. We work very closely with the radiologist. We will sometimes look at the films with the radiologist together. We get along very well."

At the end of the interview the patient said, "That's exactly what I wanted."

The wife said, "When he started getting back pain, it started messing with him psychologically and it was bothering him. He was wondering about what was going on."

Both the patient and his wife seemed extremely happy as Dr. Spangler told Dr. Atlas in front of them – he literally filled out the note with a long list of things and tests to get done before coming back in two weeks.

When Dr. Spangler got back into the charting room she said, "Nobody read the freaking paper. I go off road all the time, but you have to know why you're going off." She then made some comments about the urologist who is treating the patient at Benedict Hospital that was the only physician that they had seen – just a urologist, never the oncologist, never anyone else from radiation oncology. Again, she was referring to the fact that the patient did not get immediate hormonal therapy in the clinical setting of localized metastatic prostate cancer.

There are several important points illustrated by this vignette. First, the patient can tell the diagnosis narrative as well as anyone else because he's been socialized into the biomedical paradigm – our preferred cultural narrative. He knew the missing laboratory value, knew where to find it in his file of records that he kept, and knew how it related to the rest of his care. He referred to his diagnosis as "Stage IV." The medical system and the doctor socialized the patient into the life world of the diagnosis narrative. This is a type of persuasion to the social myth or belief system of scientific medicine. The patient said, "I'm having back pain and that worries me. I use the word 'worried'; I could use the word 'concerned.'" He then pointed to a lump in the back. The wife referred to the fact that it was bothering him "psychologically." Later, I discuss comments like these by the patient and the wife as "an existential threat." For now, it is important to realize the emotionally shared cognition by the patient is part of the diagnostic process, requiring an interim diagnosis. The patient was seeking the second opinion specifically because "they weren't aggressive enough. They haven't done any scan since my diagnosis." The issue of CT scans and re-imaging as a form of interim diagnosis is absent from the care he received and the patient understands that without the doctor telling him. Likewise, when Dr. Spangler lists all of the CT scans and imaging studies he needs and how the radiologists work closely with the oncologists, the patient summarizes, "That's exactly what I wanted."

The next vignette demonstrates the exact same thing – the patient and family are conversant in medical jargon and the language of biomedicine.

The nurse took the initial history for next patient who was an elderly gentleman; his wife accompanied him. The wife gave the entire history and was totally in control. She complained, "He's been moody for the last three months. His PSA was 2.0 at the beginning of April. He was due to get Lupron at the end of April and his prior PSA before that was 2.3 and the one before that was even higher. He's been on Lupron since July of 2011." The wife also said, "He had a negative CT scan on April 12. He sees a cancer doctor in Florida at Moffett clinic. They put him on Casodex,[7] I forgot to tell that girl. We go back to Kentucky in September and visit some friends, and then go visit my daughter in Tampa, and then go to our place in Florida where we winter." The wife actually reported the results of the CT scan done at Moffett Clinic in Florida and knew the exact date of the exam.

Outside in the charting area, Dr. Spangler was at the computer and she said to nobody in particular, "Yeah, he got a bone scan. . . . If he's having more pain he may need radiation." She then went in to see the patient.

Dr. Spangler asked the patient, "How about pain?"

The wife interrupted and said, "He is the pain." The wife was reading newspapers. She said, "I was reading in the newspapers that prostate cancer is a slow growing cancer."

Dr. Spangler then said, "Yes that was a big deal up there on Capitol Hill . . . there is a lot of controversy about unnecessary treatment. But you talk to two different people and one person will say it saved my life and the other person may say that's totally crazy. Some primary care doctors don't think we should be screening with PSA, but you have a lymph node on your CT scan."

The wife interrupted, saying, "The CT scan in Florida was negative."

Dr. Spangler continued saying, "There was all that mess about mammograms, but we got that fixed: women are better advocates. I don't agree with that PSA fear. We have it. We might as well use it." Dr. Spangler pointed out to the patient's wife, "He's been living with prostate cancer for years and that some people with pancreatic cancer or lung cancer die within a year. This seems like the reverse, but I'm going to stop the Casodex. Sometimes by stopping the medicine, it has the effect we want." She acknowledged multiple times that this was counterintuitive but then advised the patient, "Don't think about it too much." Dr. Spangler alluded to the fact that if this doesn't work that they would have to get "more aggressive."

The patient asked, "What is my PSA?"

Dr. Spangler checked, "0.7."

"So, it's higher."

Dr. Spangler replied, "At least it's less than 1.0. Everything is done by monitoring the PSA. That's very important."

"The Lupron gives me mood swings, hot flashes, and muscle aches."

Dr. Spangler acknowledged, "You have every single side effect of the therapy. It's just too bad – do it anyway. Are you buying this argument?"

The patient replied bluntly, "No."

"You have to do it anyway."

Later when we were in the charting room one of the nurses brought the issue up again and Dr. Spangler said, "His other option was an orchiectomy."[8]

In this case, the patient's wife forgot to tell the nurse that the patient was on a new hormonally active medication (Casodex), but she knew the name of the medication and when it was prescribed. She also knew the results of the CT scan. Dr. Spangler said, "You have a lymph node on your CT scan," and the wife corrected her saying, "The [subsequent] CT scan in Florida was negative." The patient himself is asking for an update by using the words, "What is my PSA?" He understands this number is a reflection of his disease progression – the amount of pain he is experiencing represents something else. Again, the participation by the patient is so complete that the patient and the doctor understand the disease process in the same way.

The following example demonstrates how the patient tries to exist in the world of the doctor, but seems to be his own worst enemy. His multiple concerns result in confusion in testing, diagnosis, and treatment. He confuses a symptom with a diagnosis. The middle of the interview with the nurse practitioner demonstrates multiple miscommunications and evidence where the conversation has major disconnects, such as when the patient confuses the bronchoscope with the gastroduodenoscopy, both abridged to "scope." The son gets frustrated and interrupts the conversation with the nurse practitioner, asking for Dr. Spangler. Yet, the patient and his family are very well socialized into the world of prostate cancer therapy and the relationship to following the PSA as a marker of disease.

Dr. Spangler and Jane[9] were chatting about the very last patient of the morning, even though it was 12:30 in the afternoon. Dr. Spangler picked up the chart and started going over labs in the computer. She looked at the flowsheet and printed reports. The nurse practitioner picked up the chart, looked at the labs, and printed papers and reports, and then the nurse practitioner went into see the patient. The first thing the patient wanted to know, of course, was his lab results. The nurse practitioner said it was 0.1 and instantaneously the patient, patient's son, and the patient's wife all broke into to very broad smiles, relaxed, and were extremely happy. The son said, "That's good, because it was 0.3 last time. Of course we wanted to be < 0.02."

The nurse practitioner said, "It takes time."

The patient probably had been waiting for three hours. Everyone seemed exhausted. The nurse practitioner asked him, "When was your colonoscopy? The gastroenterologist ordered a CT scan of the abdomen but you haven't had it yet. You should get an upper endoscopy to screen for cancer – I mean, ulcers."

The patient said, "So ulcers?"

The nurse practitioner said, "Yes, ulcers . . . or reflux."

The patient asked, "Does the lung doctor do the scope?"

The nurse practitioner said, "No, the lung doctor does PFTs, the G.I. doctor does the scope."[10]

At that point, the son said, "Are you going to bring Dr. Spangler now?"

I was standing there in the documentation room. Dr. Spangler came in and said, "Okay let's get rid of that last patient. He doesn't have that many questions right?"

The nurse practitioner said, "He's got a lot of questions."

The medical assistant came in and said, "He's chomping at the bit."

Dr. Spangler went in and apologized for being late. The patient, the patient's son, and the patient's wife were absolutely delighted and smiling to see Dr. Spangler. Very shortly, they started talking and laughing again. They repeated, "We want the PSA to be zero." The patient kept throwing out concerns and symptoms, none of which seemed to be addressed during this office visit. He again mentioned bloating and nausea. He said, "I'm losing weight because I don't want to eat."

Dr. Spangler said, "Your sodium is 131. Maybe that's because you aren't eating. Thank goodness you have a primary care doctor. He can go try and sort all these things out."

"My gastroenterologist questions the diagnosis of Crohn's disease."

Dr. Spangler said, "Maybe the nausea is from the Crohn's disease."

The son said, "No, he was not suspecting Crohn's disease as a possible explanation for his gastrointestinal symptoms."

Dr. Spangler replied, "Wait a minute, he can't take back a diagnosis. I think you should have an upper endoscopy. I can call the gastroenterologist so that they know what's going on."

The patient asked, "Is the nausea not related to the cancer?"

"It's not related to cancer," and once again big smiles all the way around the room. They were all very happy with that.

Again, "It's not related to the cancer" brings out smiles all around. As in the previous example, the patient, the doctor and the patient's family are all using a common language related to the diagnosis. This is the "re-education" W.H.R. Rivers referred to and the "learning through the other" by the process of "joint attention" to the diagnosis narrative described by Michael Tomasello.

The diagnosis narrative is only effective if the patient can recognize the diagnosis story as the story of the disease affecting themselves. Achieving joint attention between the doctor and the patient to the diagnostic narrative is a key component of the clinical encounter because it is necessary to move from diagnosis to therapy or treatment. If the patient is not persuaded – a narrative failure – then the process ends without benefit. I will describe such a case later. Once the persuasion occurs and therapy is performed, the patient is fully integrated into the experience and based on that experience can begin to use the diagnosis to narrate the story of their disease. To do this, the patient learns the language of the diagnosis and medical jargon. Metaphorically, the doctor and the patient "are on the same page" of the story. The distinction between the diagnosis narrative and the illness narrative blurs as the story becomes shared between the doctor and the patient. Mattingly and others describe this as the "preferred narrative," the one with social power. This story is the one that can lay claim on society's resources. As mentioned in the discussion of theory, the story precedes the experience (a diagnostic schema) and the experience of the diagnosis and therapy can be narrated (the diagnosis narrative), just as Jerome Bruner, Mattingly, and others described.

Notes

1　Renal is a word to describe the kidney.
2　During CT scans or MRIs a contrast dye is injected into the vein. First it is collected in the tissue of the kidney, and second it concentrates into the collecting system (the plumbing), making it easier to identify anatomical structures.
3　Images created by taking slices at a ninety-degree angle for the entire length of the body – starting at the side of the body and moving toward the middle.
4　Most common angle of slices – through the body as if it were a sausage.
5　Compact disc.
6　Lupron is a trade name for a hormonal anti-androgen treatment.
7　Casodex is the brand name for bicalutamide, a medication that binds to the androgen receptor, blocking the effect of testosterone; it is a treatment for prostate cancer.
8　An orchiectomy is a surgical procedure to remove the testicles – castration.
9　Jane is a registered nurse, but functioned as a medical assistant for Dr. Spangler, evaluating each patient before being seen by Dr. Spangler.
10　PFTs means pulmonary (lung) function tests.

Reference

Mattingly, Cheryl. 1998. *Healing Dramas and Clinical Plots: The Narrative Structure of Experience*. Cambridge: Cambridge University Press.

8   Spatial therapy

From diagnosis to therapy and diagnosis within therapy

This next vignette illustrates the relationship of diagnosis to therapy when Dr. Jeffries says, "I need a couple of days so I can get an operative plan in my head and counsel him appropriately. . . . How about Friday afternoon? . . . That's when we were thinking about doing surgery." Dr. Jeffries is describing aloud the cognitive process of taking a three-dimensional diagnosis and converting it into action, converting it into surgical therapy. Another fascinating aspect of this vignette occurs when he reverts to looking at the CT scan images despite having his hands inside the patient's body and visualizing the surgical field through a laparoscope. He depends on his cognitive hologram of the diagnosis narrative to the extent that it overrides his perceptual senses of touch, feel, and vision. The vignette starts in the office reviewing the CT scan and proceeds to the operating room in what turned out to be one of the more difficult surgeries during my fieldwork.

Dr. Jeffries was reviewing a CT scan and looking at hepatic veins. (I knew that because he was talking to himself and he said it aloud to himself.) He then turned to Dr. Stein and said, "What you think about this?" Dr. Jeffries was sitting at the bar stool on the far left computer with his screen and Dr. Stein leaned over, put his arm on the back of the chair and the two of them were simultaneously looking at the CAT scan. They reviewed the entire scan again looking at a tumor in the kidney and then some shadowing hepatic veins. Dr. Jeffries said, "Here. Here's the coronals. . . . This is why I am concerned."

Dr. Stein said, "That looks like CT contrast." His opinion was the shadow that Dr. Jeffries was looking at was contrast and he took his hand away from Dr. Jeffries's chair saying, "You might be right." He was referring to possible growth of the tumor into the hepatic veins.

Dr. Jeffries said, "Would you get an MRI?"

Dr. Stein replied, "Hell, yeah. You want to know that before you get in there."

The morning drifted into the afternoon clinic session. Dr. Stein said to Dr. Jeffries something about the free lunch from the pharmaceutical representative and then in a discreet voice said, "You're in charge of reading the CT. It doesn't matter what the radiologist said."

Continuing the discussion, Dr. Jeffries said, "The cardiologist will not allow the patient to come off aspirin because he has a bare metal stent [in his coronary artery]. This will be my first freaking nephrectomy with 325 mg of aspirin."[1]

Dr. Stein inquired, "Are you going to do it laparoscopically?"

"Yes."

Later in the day, Dr. Jeffries was on the phone and said, "I need a couple of days so I can get an operative plan in my head and counsel him appropriately. . . . How about Friday afternoon? . . . That's when we were thinking about doing surgery."

The case transitions from the outpatient clinic to the operating room. This surgery was a "partial open laparoscopic[2] surgery," which meant that they made a six-inch curvilinear incision in the lower abdomen, just large enough to insert a hand and arm into the patient's abdomen. Just prior to the surgery, the residents were anticipating the procedure and said, "He's on aspirin."

One of the medical students asked, "Why use a scope? What's the advantage?" Dr. Wright[3] said, "The incision is smaller and easier. Dr. Jeffries does a lot of hand-assist surgery. An open surgery is much larger incision. And the patient is obese. It's really tough because it's so deep down in there," acknowledging that an obese patient would be difficult to do with hand-assist surgery anyway.

When we got to the operating room, this all became clear. There was a laparoscope inserted higher in the abdomen. A gloved right hand was visible on the flat-panel monitors hanging from the ceiling. The gloved hand was that of Dr. Pinder, the resident who started the case. He was also holding the laparoscope in his left hand and it displayed the image on the flat-panel monitor. On the flat-panel monitor, you could see Dr. Pinder's fingers grasping, pulling, and he was using the cautery attached to the laparoscope to snip tissue. Dr. Pinder could actually see his own right hand displayed about eight feet away from where his actual hand was located. He could also see the image of the laparoscope that he was manipulating with his left hand. He used this virtual image to perform the surgery. They did the entire procedure this way; there was no direct visualization of the operating field. Dr. Jeffries was talking about some part of the procedure and pointing at the screen with his index finger trying to coach and guide Dr. Pinder. Dr. Jeffries then told Dr. Pinder, "Lift things up with your hand, right up there in the corner." They were working simultaneously with forceps, cautery,[4] and feeling tissue with their fingertips. I looked up. I could see Dr. Pinder's entire hand on the screen, meaning his entire hand was inside the patient's abdomen. It soon became obvious that this was going to be a difficult surgery, so Dr. Jeffries took over from Dr. Pinder and called for help.

Dr. Jeffries announced, "We're going to use up a load of staples on this guy. We can't have him bleeding."

"There are seven staples in each stapler, and there are only two available."

Dr. Jeffries said sarcastically, "Nice. Thanks guys." At this point, they had a cloth sponge in the abdominal cavity trying to stop some of the bleeding.

At one point in the procedure, Dr. Jeffries was feeling between his thumb and his index finger, compressing the tissue and then there was an episode where Dr. Pinder was cutting tissue between Dr. Jeffries's fingers. At a certain point, Dr. Bridge entered the room. He helped identify the anatomy displayed on the monitor screens throughout the operating room. These screens were the only way anyone, including the surgeon, could see anything because the incisions were only large enough to put an instrument or a hand into the patient's body. The case was tedious and obviously risky. Dr. Jeffries was using the cautery and said, "I haven't found my ureter yet."

There was country music playing in the operating room. Dr. Bridge said, "The problem you have is the music. You should have classical music. This music is getting everyone excited."

Dr. Jeffries said, "You can change it or turn it off; it doesn't bother me. Put on some [then he named a musical artist]. Your heart's not going 120 beats per minute" [implying his was].

Dr. Bridge said, "I think you're in the right plane Jeffries.[5] Absolutely that's the right plane," and then he pointed to the screen with his index finger all the way across the room – approximately 15 to 20 feet. He cupped his hands and swung his arm indicating that Dr. Jeffries should dissect the tissue with his hands that were in the patient. Because this gesture was non-verbal and everyone in the room was fixated on the video monitors, no one other than me saw him do this.

Dr. Stephens[6] entered the room. Dr. Jeffries said to Dr. Stephens, "This is a nightmare – I thought it would be easier, but it's harder."

"Is the aspirin a problem?" Dr. Stephens inquired.

Dr. Jeffries said, "Not so far. You should have a stapler prepared." Simply observing, I was feeling and sensing the danger in the room. Dr. Jeffries was struggling.

There were eight doctors staring at the screen. They seemed mesmerized by the flat-panel monitor video images. Dr. Jeffries said, "This stuff is rock-hard. It's stuck to this flipping kidney. It doesn't look like anything other than straightforward on the CT."

The tall medical student, Dr. Bridge, Dr. Stephens, and the short medical student were all looking at a laptop computer screen of the CT images as well as the monitor on the ceiling, comparing the CT images to the video images intra-operatively. Aware of them, Dr. Jeffries said, "What are the Illuminati saying in the back of the room there?" Jeffries went on to say, "I have the whole kidney here in my hand – not the whole kidney the lower pole."

Dr. Stephens said, "Can you feel the vessels there?"

Dr. Jeffries said, "Is the CT still up? Bring it up because I want to see where the hilum[7] is."

Dr. Stephens said, "Lateral to your middle finger is okay."

Dr. Jeffries said, "Am I going to cause ischemia?" Dr. Jeffries and Dr. Stephens were discussing the case. Dr. Fields walked into the room and now all eight members of the urology team were in this one single operating room. Dr. Jeffries then said, "It gets all stuck like this. I don't want to de-vascularize the kidney."

Dr. Wright was looking at the CT, saying, "It almost seems as if those are the renal veins." Dr. Stephens and Dr. Wright were looking at the CT images displayed on the laptop computer, comparing them to the video images of the surgery. This was the same CT scan that Dr. Jeffries had pondered over earlier in the week, preparing for this surgery.

Dr. Jeffries had scrubbed in and was in a sterile gown so he held his hands up in the air, leaving the operating table, and walked over to the laptop to look at the CT scan on the computer. Dr. Stephens said, "There are two arteries."

Dr. Stephens was showing the CT scan to Dr. Jeffries who was studying the CT scan, "Where's the second artery? Behind both veins? I think this is the two veins." He then went back to the operating room table. Looking from screen to screen, Dr. Jeffries said, "[referring to an anatomical structure] – he's the issue. How do I deal with this guy? I'm open to suggestions. How do I preserve that? Something bad is all I think about."

Dr. Stephens said, "It looks like you had your fingers on the aorta."

This vignette demonstrates how important this three-dimensional cognition is to both diagnosis, but also to actual patient care. Having the surgeon's fingers on the aorta implies that the wall of the aorta can tear – a lethal consequence. The residents all sensed that their leader was engaged in a high-risk surgery. The tension in the room was palpable. The social cues to this socially engaged emotion was having multiple senior attending surgeons all giving opinions about what to do. This is unusual. I believe it reflects the inherent dangers associated with this case. The drama, according to Cheryl Mattingly, occurs when something really matters. The drama is communicated by the display emotions during the surgery (Fessler 1999). Although field notes may not convey a sense of the palpable emotions in the operating room, the "high anxiety" was unmistakable; anthropologically, I could have written the field notes as a series of display emotions. To the extent that the reader could recognize the tension and danger in the preceding story, the emotion became part of the narrative of this patient's surgery. I was interested in the perspectives of various participants in this drama, so about a week later, I asked Dr. Jeffries about his experience. He said, "I was sweating bullets. That still gives me nightmares." I asked Dr. Stephens about his experience during this surgery. He said, "It was sort of hard, being the new attending and trying to help the well-established expert. I eventually took over the case, and we were able to complete the surgery. It was sort of weird." The day after the surgery, I visited the patient while he was recovering in the hospital. Although I tried desperately to get an illness narrative from him, his only comment was, "[Dr. Jeffries] told me he got all the cancer. If he did, that's good. If he didn't, well, then that's the end of me." For the patient, cutting out cancer successfully meant averting death and all the cultural meanings associated with death. The patient's minimalist "illness narrative" was to cure his cancer; the doctor had to cut it out.

3-D diagnosis, 3-D therapy in radiation oncology

Earlier I described how Dr. Rivers was responsible for outlining the diseased organs on the CT scan before the "planner" could design a treatment plan specifically related to the three-dimensional diagnosis. The topic in this chapter is how the diagnosis determines therapy. This is just as true in radiation oncology as it is in urology. The radiation machine itself has a mini CT scan built into it. It is not a high resolution CT for diagnosis but actually takes a CT scan of the patient's position on the table to compare to the CT scan used for treatment planning. Dr. Rivers said:

> Sometimes we have to make 3 mm or 4 mm adjustments. This screen shows both the positioning CT scan and the diagnostic CT scan layered over each other. On a left to right basis we can match up the patient's position on the table to make sure that the contours match up perfectly with the planning that was done on the diagnostic CT. We match the position of the patient for each treatment with the planning CT. Sometimes there are markers placed in the organs themselves. That is another way to line up the CT images with radiation machine. Here's a gold marker for a prostate cancer case. Dr. Stein put the markers in the prostate in the biopsy suite for this case.

The next vignette highlights the spatial relationships in therapy:

> I then wandered into the control room and the technologist running the radiation therapy said, "We line the patient up and check very closely the distance from the skin to the machine. We use laser beams to match the patient's tattoos." This was in addition to the CT image that Dr. Rivers had shown me earlier. There were two helpers in the room positioning the patient, and after the patient was positioned correctly, the control room could move the machine, rotating in multiple different planes from different angles. Again, in the design and treatment planning there is a window of radiation that could be seen on the computers in the control room. There is also an intercom and double video screens you can watch the patient from two different angles and talk to the patient. The control room also had five flat-panel computer screens

all lined up on the countertop. The one on the far left had three fields displayed, the middle one was ticking as the dose was administered, the next one had the outline of the perimeter plan, the next one after that had radiologic views – again, three-dimensional radiologic views of the treatment plan – and the far right had an Excel spreadsheet with lots of numbers.

Underneath the countertop there were five large boxes (larger than a typical CPU). The person running the control room said, "These computers allow us to run all the machines."

The second patient for treatment was apparently a no-show and I was just standing there. The physicist came by and asked, "Have you seen the room yet?"

"No."

He took me into the treatment room and drew several diagrams. The table in which the patient lies is underneath the curved arm of the radiation machine. On one side of the machine is the positioning CT where they can do an ultra-quick CT of the patient to help line up with the diagnostic CT. The machine itself had a circle for where the radiation came out that could turn 360°. The arm that's arched could turn 360°. The table that was sitting on the floor could spin 360°, and so the combinations and positioning options seemed endless. The physicist showed me a stack of tungsten slabs similar to what a tool and die maker would use to trace shapes. Those all moved in and out to replicate the shape of the radiation field that is designed on the computer. "Everything is done by coordinates and turns on the four-way laser. The laser can line up all of the positioning on the radiation delivery machine, the CT scan, and the person receiving treatment. That's the isocenter image of the distance that can be projected onto the table and the patient, so this is a shadow, almost like a slide, and it's this scale, depending on where the crosshairs align, that can measure the distance from the skin to the point where the radiation is generated. This is a newer machine. It's three-dimensional alignment. It's a very cool machine." He went on to characterize his job as calibrating everything to make sure it's accurate, including the laser, the dose, and all of that. "I'm also responsible for safety of every individual in the building, monitoring how much exposure to radiation they get. I also have to check the treatment plan and sometimes test one just to make sure that the treatment plan as designed is feasible, using the equipment. Occasionally the computers do something weird – maybe 1 percent of the time." Then the physicist said something fascinating: "All of these computers talk to each other. The computers in the radiation oncology suite, and all of the computers in the control room, and the computers where they design and generate the treatment plan, and the computers in the CT scan on the arm of the radiation machine. The computers pass information one to the other to the other. The CT has to give information about the patient to the dosimetry computer and that computer has to give it to the planning computer and the planning computer has to transfer to the control room system operating room and that interfaces with those five computers and the radiation machine itself. All of this is automatic and I have to verify the system is working correctly. There's lots of computers, and everything is controlled by computer."

I emphasized the role of a three-dimensional cognition in making a diagnosis. These examples highlight the necessity of using this three-dimensional cognition to plan surgery or plan radiation therapy. Three-dimensional printing for prototypes is becoming common.

Using medical images such as CT scans, these printers can construct translucent models made with variations of acrylic resin, enabling surgeons to understand the internal structure of the livers and kidneys, such as the direction of blood vessels or the exact location of a tumor. A more realistic-looking model, made partly of polyvinyl alcohol, assimilates the wetness and texture of a real human liver, making it more suitable to cut with a surgical knife.

(Osawa 2013: B5)

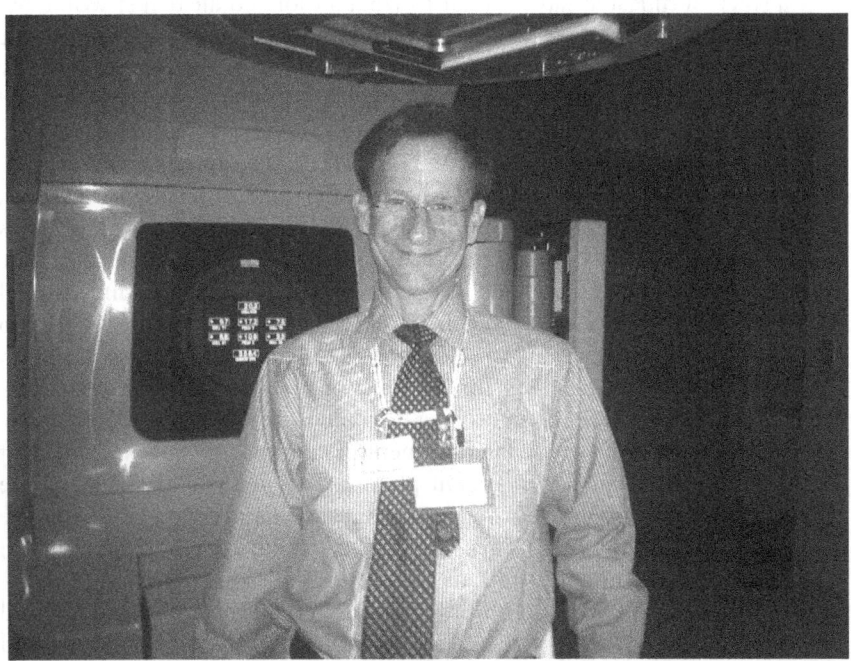

Figure 8.1 The ethnographer with laser markers for directing radiation

Although this technology is still in development, the doctors use the three-dimensional images or cognitive reconstructions for exactly the same purpose: surgical planning. Again, I would like to point out that this three-dimensional world exists within the body – a different type of spatial cognition than typically written about by anthropologists that focus on the individual in relationship to the outside world.

An ethnographic puzzle yet to be resolved

At this point in the fieldwork, I was realizing that the diagnosis narrative had a cause-and-effect relationship to the "therapeutic narrative." I recalled my original theoretical frame, the cognitive anthropology of narrative theory. In Labovian terms, the diagnosis narrative was event A and the therapeutic narrative was event B. Given the evaluative component between the two, I had my first inkling that the diagnosis narrative was a story within a story. I realized that Roy D'Andrade's concept of narrative schemas that are combined into more complex narrative schemas was a way to explain the diagnosis as the story within the more complex narrative. As I discuss the therapeutic descriptions in the ethnographic data, imagine being the ethnographer faced with the original quandary yet again: what is the narrative, who is telling the narrative? I was now on a quest to discover the more complex narrative schema. Even as I describe the exterior spatial relationship of the social field, I was cognizant of the proxemics of the story. This ethnographic hypothesis was unanswered. Typically just being there and watching, participating, and reflecting brings understanding. The next chapter tells how I resolved these questions. But first, I describe the pinnacle experience of most of the participants in this research.

Extracting the essence or object from the body

"Extracting the essence or object from the body" is the wording used by W.H.R. Rivers when he describes therapy. Consider the similarity of Quesalid's scrap of bloody feather from Claude Lévi-Strauss's *The Sorcerer and His Magic* (Lévi-Strauss 1963). Symbolically, the bloody feather is proof that the offending agent, the disease, has been removed from the body. A Da Vinci robotic prostatectomy requires omnipresent spatial relationships of the therapy in the operating room and the verbal and visual representation generated during the diagnosis narrative. Thus, therapy is an extension of diagnosis narrative – the therapeutic narrative.

The next extended excerpt is rich with correlation of the three-dimensional diagnosis and the three-dimensional therapeutics. This vignette is also included because of the importance of the Da Vinci robotic surgery to the entire urology practice and all the doctors at every stage of expertise. This is the pinnacle of biomedical competence for a urologic surgeon:

> We were in the operating room. Dr. Williamson had scrubbed in and was air-drying his hands while Dr. Stein was positioning the surgical table and asked, "Can we put this in Trendelenburg?"[8]
>
> Dr. Stein was working with the video monitor equipment. Initially the monitors were faced towards the head of the table where the anesthesiologist sat. Dr. Stein went to the back of the Da Vinci robot, and the nurse said, "You need help back there?"
>
> Dr. Stein then went to the console, which was in the corner of the room. The console connects to the robot with two large cords. Dr. Stein sat at the console, which seemed like the cockpit of a fighter jet blended with a virtual reality machine. His movements of fingers and feet controlled the surgical instruments that were inserted into the patient even though he was physically remote. Dr. Williamson was sitting on the right side near the patient's shoulder with the scrub nurse next to him and the nurse anesthetist on the other side of the drape. Dr. Williamson held a large trocar with the camera head attached to it throughout the entire procedure. He also used clips and instruments through one of the ports for this same trocar. Dr. Stein started, ensuring the micro-instruments worked properly. The scissors on the right side had an electrical current. Dr. Stein was in the console; his voice was amplified as if it was on an overhead announcer. I noticed that he was sitting and had propped the chair up so that he was looking through the double-screened slanted or angled view box. This had the appearance of old-fashioned cardboard eyeglasses from 3-D movies. These lenses were attached to the console itself. His arms were inserted underneath that, and there were foot pedals. Dr. Stein had his clogs off and he was in his sock feet. Dr. Stein verbally identified the spermatic cord and small bowel, as well as other anatomical landmarks. His voice was projected by the intercom, his eyes were looking into the console, he was controlling the robotic "arms" and using them to point to and identify the organs inside the patient's body, and multiple participants watched on multiple flat-panel monitors throughout the room. Dr. Stein and the senior resident traded turns, performing different parts of the procedure. Throughout the entire time, constant verbal interactions guided the surgical dissection as the procedure progressed.
>
> The trocars were attached to the robot that had four sliding cassettes that could go up and down; there were other parts on the robot arms that could move in space, with at least eight joints, the third one from the body of the machine was able to rotate. There were multiple instances where three or four arms were all moving simultaneously, making it look like a spider with multiple joints all moving at the same time. The arms on the robot were draped in plastic to maintain a sterile surgical field.

There were four incisions and the pneumoperitoneum insufflation[9] created an open visual field, viewable on the flat-panel monitors throughout the operating room and, of course, in the console.[10] I noticed that the right-hand was a curved scissors, and is also electrified, and often they would touch it with the outside portion of the scissors on the convex side and simply use the bovie[11] to cut away adipose tissue.

I watched the entire procedure. There was a reason patients sought out Dr. Stein; even as a non-surgeon I could tell his expert skill level. I noticed that the "hands" of the robot were interacting in terms of pulling something up, grasping it transferring it from left hand to right hand. Crossing the midline like this is a very sophisticated neurologic phenomenon and is a significant milestone in the growth and development for children. I noticed that they were able to do it here using the robot itself.

The trocars were operated by the Da Vinci robot for multi-functional surgical techniques. They could rotate, they could flip up and down, they could open, they could close, and obviously the entire trocar could change directions. Dr. Stein instructed Dr. Williamson, "Down like this but not straight like that." He was indicating angles and Dr. Williamson inserted and clamped with a plastic clamp twice. They were essentially collaborating to proceed with the surgery. After the prostate was completely dissected, Dr. Stein used one of the instruments inserted through the incision made by the trocar to grab it with both cut sections of the vas deferens[12] and hold it up into the open space inside the abdominal cavity. These were essentially embedded in the prostate.

There was a double needle on one wire suture. They started stitching. Dr. Stein went back and forth suturing the proximal urethra to the bladder neck.[13] At this point it was like shoelaces and everything was loose. He put four stitches in the proximal urethra and the bladder neck, and then said. "That will be enough where it won't back out," and he started tightening the suture like tightening shoelaces, and the back wall of the proximal urethra approximated the bladder perfectly.

Dr. Stein instructed Dr. Williamson, "Cut this one," and the needle was then passed from forceps to forceps and taken out of the abdominal cavity through the plastic trocar sheath exit. Dr. Stein started doing surgical knots, square knots, tying it the metallic suture with one needle on and the other end of bare suture.[14] The knots were perfectly tied. Dr. Stein came over and sat back down next to me and started typing on his laptop. I had previously tried to explain my thinking about space, time, and three-dimensionality, and he always acted as if he didn't understand. In this case, he told me to go over to the console and take a peek through the 3-D glasses, which I did. I went over to the console where I could see the three-dimensionality of the surgical field as if I had binocular vision in an open incision. *AMAZING!* It was like virtual reality and I was actually *inside the patient's abdomen!* This experience had a profound

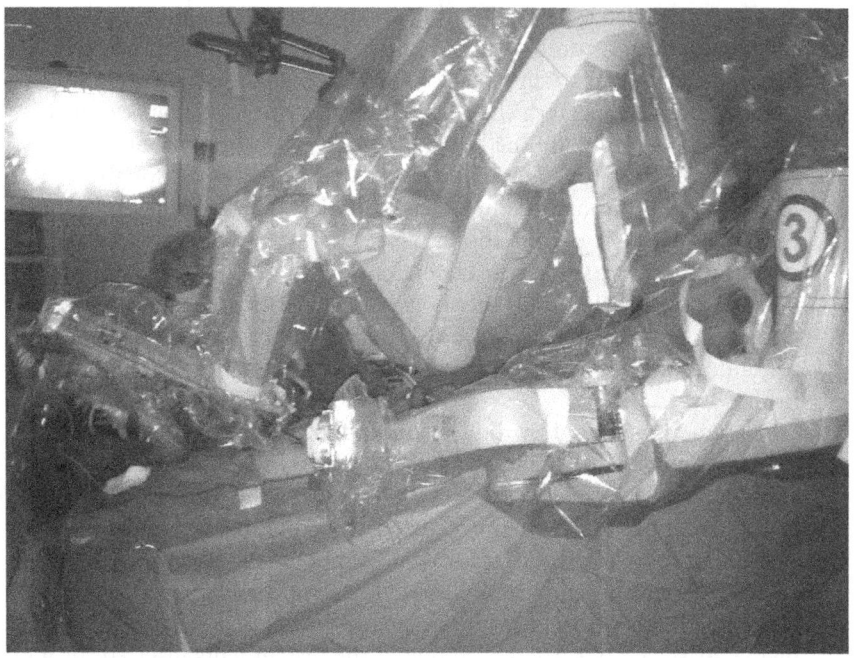

Figure 8.2 Da Vinci robotic surgical system

effect on me – I had spent hundreds of hours staring at CT and MRI scans, but this technology recreated *Fantastic Voyage* (Fleischer 1966). I did look down at the hand controls. There were actually small bands for the thumb and forefinger as you grasped the bar with again multiple joints on the arms in the console.

The three-dimensional diagnosis and chemotherapy

One could argue that the emphasis on spatial relationships and three-dimensional imaging is an artifact of my data being from surgically oriented specialties. Oncology is a specialty of internal medicine, which typically is conceptualized as heavily dependent on laboratory data. My fieldwork data showed that there was always a residual emphasis on CT imaging as the final arbiter of "removal of the disease."

Dr. Spangler said, "Are you doing a CT scan? When was the last one?" One of the residents replied, "One million years ago."

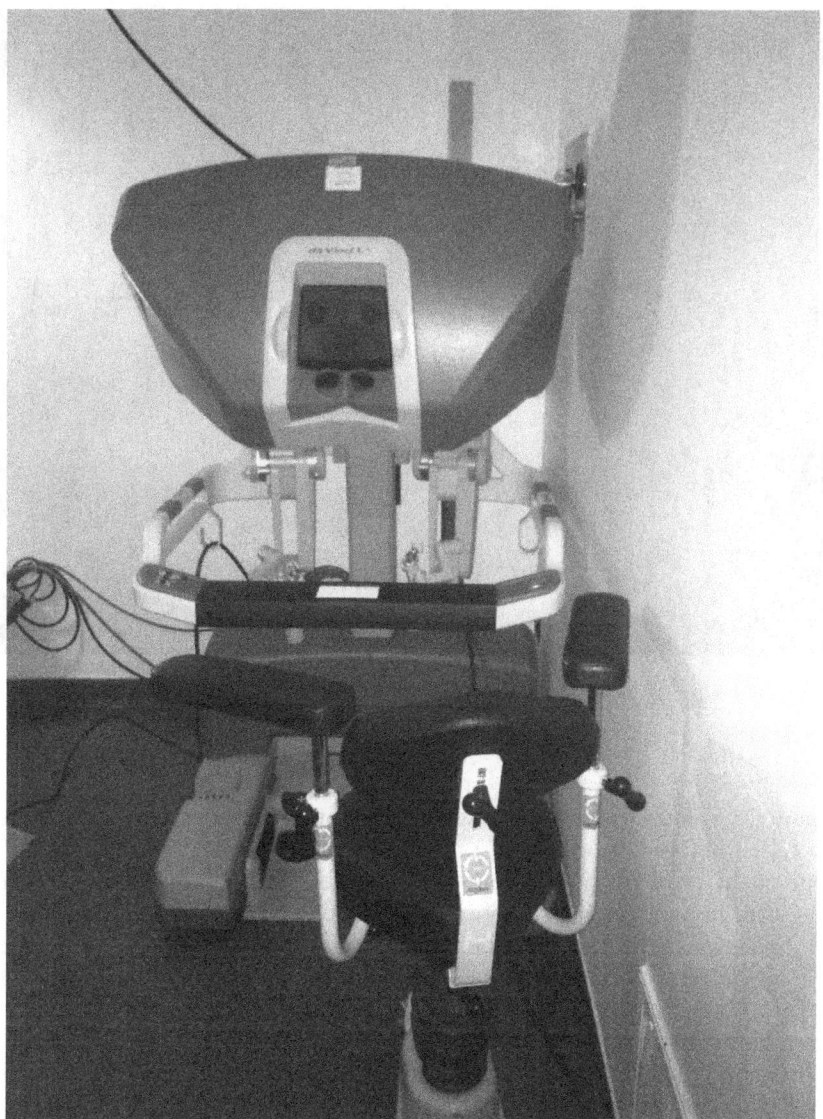

Figure 8.3 Da Vinci console

Dr. Spangler asked, "We didn't do one this admission?"
They decided they needed to do one. But they needed a reason to order it,
    not just because it's been a long time.
The resident said, "You could say we're looking for obstruction."

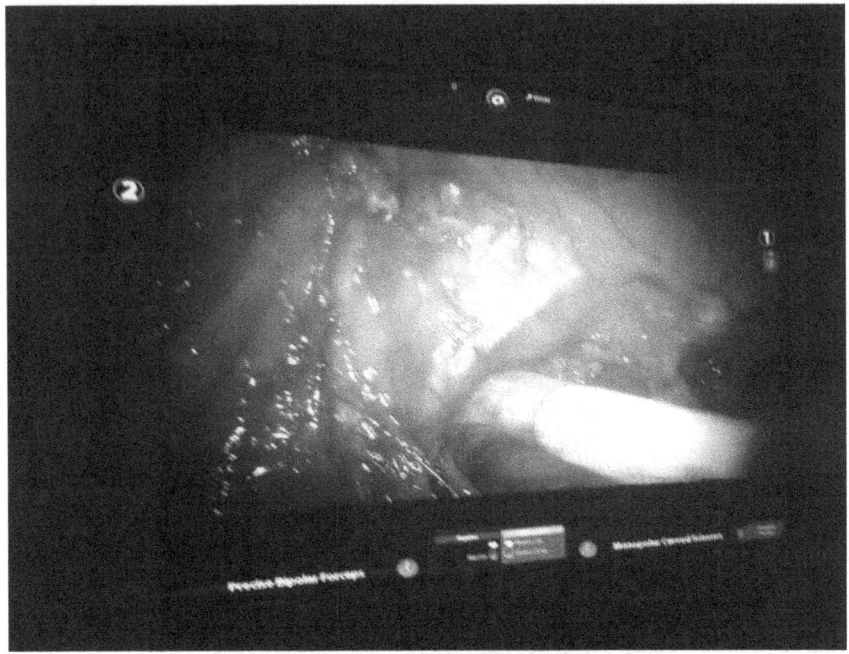

Figure 8.4 Flat-panel view with micro-instrument inside the abdomen

Again Dr. Spangler said, "When was the last one? He needs a CT scan of the chest before he goes."

One of the residents pointed out that the patient's creatinine was up. "We want to avoid giving IV contrast and extend the hospitalization."

Dr. Spangler said, "Just get a non-contrast CT because we need to get the big picture in order to treat his cancer."

Even though chemotherapy is a medication and not a surgery, a three-dimensional image is required to monitor disease progress and to guide the therapy. Every medical student takes gross anatomy and learns the three-dimensional nature of organs and diseased organs. Using a stethoscope and physical examination is another way that doctors conceptualize the three-dimensionality of disease – even for medical problems such as heart failure or pneumonia. Because the field site was a surgical subspecialty, the importance of three-dimensional cognition was easier to see, but even general practitioners have to think three-dimensionally.

The diagnostic narrative determines the etiology of the disease. That same narrative determines the correct therapy. Consider what a disaster it would be if the diagnosis narrative told the wrong story – the therapy would be the wrong therapy. The clinical encounter proceeds by removing the diseased organ from the body. This process is closely connected to the diagnosis, which guides the doctor and the patient through therapy. Again, I faced the ethnographic quandary of discovering the overarching narrative. Convinced of the veracity of the diagnosis narrative in healing practices, I turned toward another anthropological heuristic to understand the social spaces surrounding the diagnostic narrative. I was confident that my observations thus far were correct, but I lacked a complete understanding. I was still committed to using narrative theory, but the next chapter discusses how I adapt "tried and true" anthropological tools to gain new perspectives on narrative that resolved my ethnographic dilemma.

Notes

1 A stent is a wire mesh that keeps the coronary artery open, or patent. In this case, the stent is not coated with a drug to prevent clots, which means the aspirin is necessary to prevent clots.
2 A laparoscope is a tube, about a half inch in diameter, inserted through a small incision that allows visualization of the surgical area as well as insertion of small instruments to do the actual surgery.
3 Dr. Wright is a resident physician, one of the more senior residents.
4 Cautery is burning to prevent bleeding from small blood vessels such as capillaries. In this case the burn is caused by an electrical current. At other times, it is a chemical burn. Electrical cautery is also referred to as a "bovie."
5 Dr. Bridge is an emeritus professor with lots of experience. Although Dr. Bridge is still surgically active, Dr. Jeffries is the busy, active surgeon using the latest techniques.
6 Dr. Stephens is a junior faculty – he just finished his robotic surgery fellowship, a type of extra post-graduate training that allows for knowledge that is even more specialized and additional skill development.
7 The hilum is the only place the kidney is connected to the rest of the body. It contains vital anatomical structures, such as the renal artery, renal vein, and so forth.
8 A term referring to positioning of the body with the head down and the legs elevated. In this case, the patient's legs were also in stirrups, spread apart similar to a female pelvic exam.
9 This word means that the surgeons poked a hole into the abdomen and used pressurized gas to blow the interior up like a balloon. This allows a clear visual field to identify all the anatomical structures.
10 Pneumoperitoneum is air in the abdominal cavity. Insufflation means to inflate a cavity, similar to inflatable lawn entertainment systems.
11 An instrument to cauterize blood vessels to stop bleeding during surgery.
12 The vas deferens are the tubular structures that carry sperm from the testicles, through the scrotum, and penetrate the prostate before emptying into the prostatic urethra, the channel where urine comes out of the bladder.
13 This means that the prostate had been totally removed and the two loose ends of the "plumbing" were being put back together.
14 Suture is a fancy word for string, often made of very special materials for different surgical purposes.

References

Fessler, D. 1999. Toward an Understanding of the Universality of Second Order Emotions. *In Biocultural Approaches to the Emotions.* A. L. Hinton, ed. Cambridge: Cambridge University Press.

Fantastic Voyage, 1966. Feature film. Directed by Fleischer, R.

Lévi-Strauss, C. 1963. The Sorcerer and His Magic. *Structural Anthropology*, 167–185.

Osawa, J. 2013. Next to Use 3-D Printing: Your Surgeon. *Wall Street Journal*, April 9, 2013, p. B5.

Part III

Ritual healing in Western medicine

9 Ritual theory

Rituals as shared experience-narratives

I started this research using narrative theory. Illness narratives dominate narrative healing theory in the anthropological canon. Anthropological writings focus on the patient narrating a life story, striving for coherence and patching disruptions or breaches, sometimes describing a co-constructed narrative and at other times portraying the doctor as the villain (Frank 1995: 127; Greenhalgh 2001). My ethnographic data does not support such a model that is so patient-centric that it allows for the impression that doctors are peripheral to healing. I believe the discrepancy is methodological. I observed the social practices of patients and doctors interacting with each other, making the doctor present in the data. This is quite different from an anthropologist interviewing a patient in some other social space.

As mentioned in the chapter on methods, I pondered the themes brought out by coding the data. It was my insight into diagnosis narratives determining therapy that reminded me of another portion of the anthropological canon – ritual healing. The similarities between my data and ritual studies were striking. The ethnographic data presented so far supports the following labels:

1   Constructing a diagnostic narrative
2   Telling the diagnostic story to the patient
3   Joint attention to the diagnostic narrative
4   Patients are socialized to live within the world of the medical diagnosis
5   Therapy is based on the diagnostic narrative.

Reviewing the coded data themes, I recognized other important concepts related to healing rituals:

1   Patients experience disease as an existential threat
2   Patients and doctors hope for a cure
3   There is a connection between hierarchy and competence among doctors.

I tried to confirm this analysis by exploring anthropological literature on ritual healing. Previous anthropological work focused on the symbolic or mythical elements of ritual healing. I had no need to do that because the researcher (me), my readers, and the participants all share a fundamental sense of biomedicine as ideology or shared cultural myth, negating the need to explore symbolism.

The relationship between narrative and ritual

I struggled theoretically with how ritual and narrative are related. I used Tomasello's theory of the mind and the ability for joint attention to an object in the social space (such as a narrative) and looked specifically for that joint attention to a diagnosis narrative in early anthropological writing on healing rituals. It was not hard to find – it practically jumped out at me. I also looked back at writings on recent descriptions of narrative healing and to my amazement, I realized both Kleinman and Mattingly mentioned ritual, but didn't expand on how narrative and ritual are inter-related.

Every ritual is a story. Rituals use words, actions, symbols, and experiences to retell a culturally authorized myth. Recall during my discussion of the self there was a tension: which came first, the narrative or the experience? Rituals are symbolic stories that pre-exist and are simultaneously re-experienced by participants. I simply expand Tomasello's concept from two conspecifics to a group of conspecifics all experiencing a story as it unfolds in real life, one that bonds them together. Recall that I have previously documented multiple individuals, either at the clinic or in the operating room, all jointly attending to the CT images.

I expand the line of investigation started by Mattingly that healing can be described by the narrative structure of experience (Mattingly 1998: 2). However, think back to Labov's seminal definition of narrative – telling the other of an experience. This theoretical leap to experienced narratives in the form of rituals has been hinted at by Kleinman and Mattingly, but never developed. I believe "healing experience-narratives" in the form of *healing rituals* is a neglected form of "narrative healing." Theoretically, I explored the concept of healing experience-narratives and found that my data supported such a perspective.

At this point in my fieldwork, I reviewed what I knew about healing rituals and then re-examined my fieldwork data, seeking to confirm or deny this new heuristic. I found a consistent structure for healing rituals discussed by many anthropologists; I realized that the clinical encounters of Western medicine follow this same structure. At this point, I explicate what we know about ritual healing and then specifically use my ethnographic data to demonstrate concordance of what I was observing with the anthropological canon related to ritual healing. I identified the following components of healing rituals:

(1) Patients experience disease as an existential threat, creating the liminality of being unable to perform their social roles (yet to be described)

(2) Explicating the cause of disease (the diagnosis narrative)
(3) Persuasion to the preferred narrative (joint attention to the diagnosis narrative)
(4) The diagnostic narrative determines the appropriate therapy (diagnosis determines therapy)
(5) Qualifications of a "leech" (yet to be described).

I tried to confirm my conceptualization of medical clinical encounters as rituals and realized I had already described (2), (3), and (4). I had to re-examine my data and further explore both (1) and (5), which follow in the next chapters. Having such a strong concordance with my own data to the structure of healing rituals in other cultures, I argue that the modern Western clinical encounter is a healing ritual. This emergent heuristic is entirely consistent with my original theoretical frame that blended cognitive anthropology and narrative theory. This expanded theoretical frame allows for a more accurate interpretation of my data.

Rituals are enacted stories

Rituals combine pre-existing narrative in the form of myth, the experience of enacting a ritual, and a very specific structure as outlined earlier. The ritual does not work if not performed correctly. It was not hard for me to understand the social structure of healing rituals as a narrative schema. Experiencing and "telling" the story as a healing ritual is a cultural practice. The existential threat creates the drama of the narrative. The liminality of being diseased allows for the transformative movement from loss of social roles to reintegration in a new culturally authorized status. Unless the individual stays connected to the culture, they cannot narrate with a common language and they have no audience. The alienation of being "diseased" is therefore an existential threat to the narrating self; participation in a ritual mitigates that threat. Although each patient has a different story, it is actually the same story repeating itself. Such is the nature of a narrative schemata embedded in a healing ritual.

It is the relationship between experience and narrative – together with experience of ritual – that allows me to integrate these theoretical constructs into the *narrative-experience healing ritual*. In doing so, I extend and synthesize the work of Kleinman and Mattingly to describe a medical clinical encounter and how "healing" is produced in such a setting. First, I review the anthropological concept of ritual healing.

Healing rituals as described in the anthropological canon

I use Rivers's declaration of the universal motivation to enter into healing rituals – fear of disease and death (Rivers 2001 [1924]: 53–54). Evans-Pritchard provided a detailed description of the oracle as diagnostic tool (Pritchard 1976: 38–43). Meyer Fortes described divination (diagnosis) in healing rituals (Fortes 1987), and Victor Turner described the healing ritual for the affliction of *"Isoma"* as validation of the "diagnostic narrative" component of a healing ritual (Turner 1969). There are commonalities in the description of healing rituals, but for the purpose of explication, I give priority to Rivers, because he directly links healing rituals throughout time and around the world directly with Western biomedicine in its current form (Rivers 2001 [1924], Flexner 1910). I will next explore each component of the healing ritual as described by the aforementioned anthropologists.

James Dow also recognizes the universality of ritual healing, but he is concerned with the common structure that can describe and explain the organization of all forms of symbolic healing regardless of the culture in which healing occurs. He gives us the following:

(1) The experiences of healers and healed are generalized with culture-specific symbols in *cultural myth*.
(2) A suffering patient comes to a healer who persuades the patient that the *problem can be defined* in terms of the myth.
(3) The *healer* attaches the patient's emotions to transactional symbols particularized from the general myth.
(4) The healer *manipulates the transactional symbols* to help the patient transact his or her own emotions.

(Dow 1986: 56–69; emphasis added)

For my discussion of clinical encounters, the generalized myth is medical science, the definition of the problem is a diagnosis, and the healer uses joint attention to a diagnostic narrative as a form of persuasion. The emotion of the existential threat allows the healer to manipulate the symbols by attaching a therapeutic plan to the diagnosis (cut out the cancer). In this way, Dow's work on the common structure of the healing ritual validates ritual components that I previously described with the ethnographic data I have already presented.

Jerome D. Frank did cross-cultural work and outlined the following prerequisites of a healing ritual:

(1) A healing agent, typically a person trained in a socially sanctioned method of healing believed to be effective by the sufferer and at least some members of his or her social group.
(2) A sufferer who seeks relief from the healer
(3) A healing relationship – that is, a circumscribed, more or less structured series of contacts between the healer and the sufferer.

(Frank and Frank 1991: 2)

He goes on to describe the structure of the healing ritual:

(1) An emotionally charged, confiding relationship with a helping person
(2) A healing setting

(3) A rationale, conceptual scheme, or myth that provides a plausible expla-
     nation for the patient's symptoms and prescribes a ritual or procedure
     for resolving them
(4) A ritual or procedure that requires the active participation of both
     patient and therapist and that is believed by both to be the means of
     restoring the patient's health.

                                               (Frank and Frank 1991: 40–44)

Again, salient components of the ritual discussed in my data are a socially
sanctioned agent (the doctor), an emotionally charged relationship (the existential threat), a plausible explanation (the diagnosis), and a ritual procedure requiring participation (experienced by both) in the form of therapy
specific to the diagnosis. Note particularly that participation by both patient
and therapist is required to perform a healing ritual.

Medicine, disease, and doctors: the healing ritual

The advancement of science depends on building scientific models. Healing
rituals have a long and illustrious legacy in the discipline of anthropology,
and at this point contrasting and comparing them with my ethnographic
data will provide part of the analysis of my data. I argue that the healing
ritual in Western biomedicine is structurally and functionally the same as
healing rituals in many other diverse cultures throughout the globe.

   W.H.R. Rivers, in his book *Medicine, Magic and Religion* (2001 [1924])
provides a global perspective on a multitude of different cultures and
describes the basic elements of each. Most of the societies he surveyed were
small-scale societies. After brief discussion of magic and religion he turns to
medicine, stating:

> Medicine, on the other hand, is a term for a set of social practices by
> which man seeks to direct and control a specific group of natural phe-
> nomenon – viz. those especially affecting man himself, which so influ-
> ences behavior as to unfit him for the normal accomplishment of his
> physical and social functions – phenomenon which lower his vitality
> and tend towards death. By a process of generalization, society has
> come to classify these phenomena together, and has distinguished them
> from other groups of natural phenomena under the name of *disease*.
>
>   (Rivers 2001 [1924]: 4; emphasis added)

Notice that the disease makes the person unfit for social functions. Rivers specifically uses the term *disease*. Disease is a shared social construct,
whereas illness is individual and unique. Illnesses are not diagnosed; diseases
are. This distinction lends validity to my earliest observations related to the
diagnosis narrative. When discussing the various linguistic nomenclature
for practitioners of the healing art, Rivers chooses the term "leech" when

speaking of a member of society whose special function it is to deal with the cure of disease (Rivers 2001 [1924]: 5). Others use the words *medicine man, shaman, diviner*, or *doctor*.

One of the reasons why medicine, magic, and religion are worldwide is that "disease and death are so closely connected that, even if the earth had been divided up into independent and self-contained apartments, we should have expected much similarity in the reaction of different groups of mankind towards them" (Rivers 2001 [1924]: 54). It is important to note that the potential threat of a disease – not an illness – invokes the healing ritual. I maintain that a disease is a social construction and, as such, a shared cognition between an individual self and the cultural body. "Life and Death" stories are stories worth telling (Labov's reportability). In order to expand our knowledge about healing, I need to fill the negative space of our understanding and describe the "story of the healing ritual." The story begins with an existential threat. In my earlier work, I referred to the existential threat as a "narrative dilemma" (Meza and Passerman 2011). In hindsight, that patient told a clinical story to the doctor when the fear of death created the inability of the patient to narrate the fear of disease. This created a narrative dilemma, otherwise known as an existential threat, initiating a healing ritual.

Diagnosis narratives in ritual studies

Rivers expounds on the relationship of the causal effect described in my original discussion of narrative.

> One element of the concept of disease, and perhaps the most important, is that it includes within its scope the factor of causation. There are usually clear-cut ideas concerning the immediate conditions, which lead to the appearance of disease. One happy result of this fact is that we are able to approach our subject by way of the etiology, and are thus led to deal with the medicine of the savage peoples from the same standpoint as that of modern medicine, which rests, or should rest, entirely upon the foundation of etiology.
>
> (Rivers 2001 [1924]: 7)

Identifying the etiology of disease is otherwise known as naming the disease (diagnosis).

Notice the frequency of the term "cause," taking us back to Michael Tomasello, who described human experience as organized intentional beings who understand the world in terms of causal events, allowing the development of culture. Western medicine fits perfectly within Rivers's global survey of explanations for disease under the category of disease as a result of natural causes (biomedicine). Rivers points out that it is the "leech" (doctor) who "carries out proceedings which correspond with those we call diagnosis" by the practice of "leechcraft." I described how, in current medical practice, it is the doctor that tells the diagnosis narrative and the patient is informed, or is the recipient of the naming of the disease. This is accomplished by joint attention to the diagnosis narrative.

Bringing us close to contemporary medicine, Rivers says:

> The emergence of medicine from its intimate associations with religion and magic is closely connected with the gradual substitution of the concept of physical causation for the spiritual list of agencies of the animism which formed the early attitude towards nature. The growth of medicine is closely bound up with the development of the concept of the natural world as opposed to world we now regard as supernatural.
>
> (Rivers 2001 [1924]: 110)

He continues:

> For the worms and snakes of savage medicine have been substituted from microscopic and ultra-microscopic organisms of the germ theory of disease, while the place of the old humours has been taken by the alteration in the proper proportion of internal secretions which is now coming to be recognized as an immediate cause of so many morbid states.
>
> (Rivers 2001 [1924]: 111)

The reason for this substitution takes us back to the cognitions of causation: "Every physical event has its physical antecedent, without the presence of which it would not itself have come into existence. The progress of physical science depends largely on the robustness of the faith in this law of causation" (Rivers 2001 [1924]: 116). The diagnosis narrative as an assertion of causation serves this same essential function of ritual experience in my data set.

Evans-Pritchard, in his ethnography *Witchcraft, Oracles, and Magic Among the Azande* (1976) provides even greater detail on the diagnostic process. When a man's health is threatened, there is a highly elaborated process for finding out the etiology or cause, in this case a result of witchcraft from some other person in the society. The process of diagnosis is described as follows:

> They take a chicken to the name of one person and pour poison down its throat, and ask the poison oracle whether this man is the witch or not. If the Oracle says that this particular person has nothing to do with the health of the inquirer then they take another chicken to the name of the second person and repeat the test. When the oracle kills a fowl to a man's name, i.e., says that it is he who will cause the inquirer sickness among the coming month, they then ask it whether this is the only witch

who threatens his welfare or whether there also others in the offing. If the oracle says that there are others, then they must seek them out till the oracle says that there is no need to inquire further since he now possessed the name of all the witches will cause the Inquirer ill health.

(Pritchard 1976: 38)

Pritchard details the sequence of asking questions and confirming the answers from the oracle. The oracle asks questions both in the positive and in the negative and these need to concur. In essence, this becomes a process of diagnosing the cause of the suffering or disease (caused by witchcraft). Meyer Fortes (Fortes 1987) and Victor Turner (Turner 1969) also provide descriptions that support these same concepts.

Noting the proximity of diagnosis to therapeutics, Rivers states,

Mankind has theories of the causation of disease, carries out proceedings which correspond with those we call diagnosis and prognosis, and finally has modes of treatment which, even if they have little in common with our own remedies, nevertheless may be regarded as making up a definite system of therapeutics.

(Rivers 2001 [1924]: 6)

Later, he says,

This lesson is the rationality of the leechcraft of such peoples as the Papuan and the Melanesian. The practices of these peoples in relation to disease are not a medley of disconnected and meaningless customs, but are inspired by definite ideas concerning the causation of disease. Their modes of treatment follow directly from their ideas concerning etiology and pathology.

(Rivers 2001 [1924]: 48)

Rivers could easily have been describing a Da Vinci robotic radical prostatectomy for prostate cancer when he wrote those words. The foundation of our current cultural model: "Cancer – cut it out" is consistent with Rivers's descriptions. It is this striking concordance of this description of ritual with the ethnographic data I have already presented that convinced me I was observing healing rituals in my fieldwork.

Importantly, Evans-Pritchard also delineates the social roles that correspond to diagnosis and therapeutics: "The Azande witch doctor is both diviner and magician. As diviner he exposes witches; as magician he thwarts them" (Pritchard 1976: 66). Evans-Pritchard reinforces Rivers's link between the "diagnosis" and the treatment. Azande divining is analogous to the diagnosis narrative. Urologists used the oracle of the CT scan image and reconstituted it into a three-dimensional representation of the "health of the individual" and confirmed it with the MRI to divine that disease was present before thwarting the prostate cancer with a Da Vinci robotic prostatectomy. The Azande also have a cause-and-effect cognitive structure to the diagnostic and therapeutic process: a witch causes disease using witchcraft; the magician thwarts witchcraft using magic.

Controlling disease by joint participation in ritual healing

W.H.R. Rivers describes medicine as a set of social practices that "seek to direct and control" disease (Rivers 2001 [1924]: 4). The imperative to control disease derives from the notion that "[disease lowers] vitality and tend toward death" (Rivers 2001 [1924]: 4). Although subtle, Rivers identifies the object controlled as the disease, not the person or the body, as portrayed by Foucauldian thought. This allows for shared participation in a cultural practice, as both patient and leech agree with the basic intent of their shared activity, control of disease. Although subtle, this distinction is at odds with much of the anthropological writing that portrays doctors and biomedicine as struggling for control of the narrative. Using the heuristic of ritual, both patient and doctor form a team to defeat disease and death – death is the ultimate form of totalitarianism; death has ultimate control over both the diagnosis narrative and the illness narrative. If there was no disease or death, there would be no need for leeches (doctors) or leechcraft (medicine).

Although power is often discussed – and maligned by anthropologists in anthropological literature (Hahn 1995), power or specialized knowledge is necessary for a healing ritual. Rivers framed healing rituals as controlling disease and death, not controlling persons. Again, in these examples of ritual healing, both the "leech" and the patient are part of the cultural body. It would thus seem logical to analyze both the doctor and the patient as being the object controlled by the body politic.

Persuasion – joint attention to the diagnosis narrative

Rivers continues his formulation with multiple references to causation: "One element of the concept of disease, and perhaps the most important, is that it includes within its scope the factor of causation" (Rivers 2001 [1924]: 6) Tomasello reminds us that humans understand the world in causal terms (Tomasello 1999: 18–19). Shared cognitions of causal understanding create culture and, in this case, the subculture of Western medicine. Again, in order for medicine to be sustained as a cultural practice, it must be a shared understanding, and in this case a shared understanding between doctor and patient. Rivers says:

> In the case of one process, the attainment of self-knowledge as a means of treatment, the resemblance with the social process of normal health

is so obvious that the physician has come to use a term derived therefrom. The process by which a faulty trend of feeling, thought, or conduct is diverted into a more healthy channel is generally known as re-education.

(Rivers 2001 [1924]: 127)

In the case of the healing ritual, Rivers refers to the "re-education" of the patient into the belief system of the leech after the proper diagnosis has been ascertained (Rivers 2001 [1924]:12). If the fundamental structure of the healing ritual results in the re-education into the natural causes of the disease, this bears a marked resemblance to the endeavor of Western biomedicine. For this reason, I use Rivers's term "re-education," *persuasion*, and joint attention to the diagnostic-therapeutic narrative interchangeably. It is imperative to acknowledge that the patient is persuaded to recognize in themselves part of a culture that they implicitly share with the doctor – biomedical science. This is not a form of aggression or control of the story by the doctor against the patient. Rather, it is as James Dow described, "*The healer attaches the patient's emotions to transactional symbols particularized from the general myth.*" The emotion of terror from the existential threat is redirected to the diagnosis narrative, allowing the ritual to proceed. Even Kleinman alludes to this same process. "Re-education" is part of Kleinman's explanatory model. He says, "No doctor is taught how to explain the biomedical account to patients. Yet this is an essential task in the work of doctoring" (Kleinman 1988: 240).

Patients are socialized to live within the world of the medical diagnosis and to use that social reality to deal with ongoing disruptions in their lives. Thus, the disease and how it is "removed" becomes a part of the self-narrative, allowing for the ongoing self-narrative to continue through a transformative process that is socially recognized, supported, and sanctioned. The process of re-education creates a change in the patients' self-stories, a second major component of narrative within the healing ritual. The self-stories converge with the diagnosis narrative and become a shared *diagnosis-illness narrative*.

When observing the healing rituals, Evans-Pritchard gives the following insight: "If one witch doctor fails to cure Azande he goes to another in the same way as we go to another doctor if we're dissatisfied with the treatment of the first one we've consulted" (Pritchard 1976: 108). I will present data of patients seeking second opinions. They are following a pattern described by Evans-Pritchard. If there is a failure to agree upon the diagnosis, the healing ritual becomes a narrative failure and the individual becomes suspended in unnamed disease or disputed disease, unable to complete the ritual and the desired transformation it provides. I will present examples from my data and from the anthropological literature to illustrate this point.

Liminality in ritual

Cheryl Mattingly quotes Jerome Bruner saying,

> If narrative is based on a "breach" of the commonplace, then pro-
> found physical and mental suffering constitutes one breach that seems
> to demand a narrative shape. It is one *liminal place* [emphasis added]
> within the human condition that calls for sense-making and this often
> takes narrative form (Bruner 1986; Bruner 1996).
>
> (Mattingly 1998: 1)

The term breach, used by Bruner, is synonymous with the terms disruption,
unexpected, and, I will argue, synonymous with the term existential threat
that I use in presenting my data. A narrator tries to get to the other side of
liminality through a narrative endeavor.

Qualifications of a leech

Rivers (and others) describe another aspect of medicine that is consistent
with a biomedical healing ritual. Speaking further about the qualifications
for a leech, Rivers says:

> The most complete instruction in any branch of medical magical or
> medical religious art is of no avail to the people unless money has passed
> from himself to his instructor. This instruction and purchase, however,
> nearly always include both the production and cure of disease, where
> disease is ascribed to human agency in the power and knowledge to
> perform rights other than those of the curative nature where medicine
> is allied with religion.
>
> (Rivers 2001 [1924]: 41)

I will provide further aspects of training a leech later.
  Repeating what Rivers said, Evans-Pritchard states:

> Magic must be bought like any other property, and the really significant
> part of initiation is the slow transference of knowledge about plants
> from teacher to pupil in exchange for a long string of fees. A teacher
> may show them casually to his pupil at any time when they were both
> out in the bush together, as on a hunting trip, or he may specially take
> him out for the purpose. Unless the medicines are bought with adequate
> fees there's a danger that they will lose their potency for the recipient
> during the transference, since their owner is dissatisfied and bears the
> purchaser ill will.
>
> (Pritchard 1976: 97)

The modern-day version of that is a medical-surgical residency. There is a connection between hierarchy, experience, and competence among doctors.

Meyer Fortes also talks about training and its vital role in generating a healing ritual:

> But I have in mind more the fact that divination is often a specialized technique. The diviner may have to undergo training to become expert in it, or he may be selected for it by virtue of his talents for his psychological makeup. The diviner must be properly accredited, often by a public initiation after evidence of his acceptance by the occult agencies.
>
> (Fortes 1987: 10)

Those passages describe the initiation and transfer of the systems of meaning that constitute diagnosis and therapeutics. This is as much a part of the healing ritual as any other.

Summary

I started with narrative theory and explained how the self is necessary for narrative. I explored the inseparability of *experience* and *narrative* as being two sides of the same coin. I discovered that illness narratives are not part of clinical encounters I observed. I described diagnosis narratives and their relationship to therapeutics. Because of these findings, I re-analyzed my ethnographic data to verify that current clinical encounters in Western medicine follow standard structures of healing rituals. I firmly believe these are interrelated concepts. I intend to show this interrelationship as I describe healing experience-narratives as a form of ritual.

References

Bruner, Jerome. 1986. *Actual Minds, Possible worlds*. Cambridge, MA: Harvard University Press.

———. 1996. *The Culture of Education*. Cambridge, MA: Harvard University Press.

Dow, James. 1986. Universal Aspects of Symbolic Healing: A Theoretical Synthesis. American Anthropologist. *New Series* 88(1):56–69.

Flexner, Abraham. 1910. *Medical Education in the United States and Canada*. New York: The Carnegie Foundation for the Advancement of Teaching.

Fortes, Meyer. 1987. *Religion, Morality, and the Person: Essays on Tallensi Religion*. Cambridge: Cambridge University Press.

Frank, Arthur W. 1995. *The Wounded Storyteller: Body, Illness, and Ethics*. Chicago: University of Chicago Press.

Frank, Jerome D., and Julia B Frank. 1991. *Persuasion & Healing: A Comparative Study of Psychotherapy*. Baltimore: Johns Hopkins University Press.

Greenhalgh, Susan. 2001. *Under the Medical Gaze*. Berkeley: University of California Press.

Hahn, Robert A. 1995. *Sickness and Healing*. New Haven, CT: Yale University Press.

Kleinman, Arthur. 1988. *The Illness Narratives – Suffering, Healing, and the Human Condition*. New York: Basic Books.

Mattingly, Cheryl. 1998. *Healing Dramas and Clinical Plots: The Narrative Structure of Experience*. Cambridge: Cambridge University Press.

Meza, James, and Daniel Passerman. 2011. *Integrating Narrative Medicine and Evidence-Based Medicine: The Everyday Social Practice of Healing*. New York: Radcliffe.

Pritchard, E., and E. Evans. 1976. *Witchcraft, Oracles, and Magic Among the Azande*. Oxford: Clarendon Press.

Rivers, W.H.R. 2001 [1924]. *Medicine, Magic, and Religion*. London: Routledge Classics.

Tomasello, Michael. 1999. *The Cultural Origins of Human Cognition*. Cambridge, MA: Harvard University Press.

Turner, Victor. 1969. *The Ritual Process*. Chicago: Aldine.

10 Disease as an existential threat

Existential threats in medicine

In my discussion of ritual as experienced narrative, W.H.R. Rivers emphasized heavily the "existential threat" of disease and death. If my analysis is correct, I should find evidence of such existential threats in my data. Again, I did not have to look hard – they were easy to see.

Disease is the natural cause of death and is experienced as an existential threat to the body in the form of the death of the body. In the next scenario, I would like to expand *existential threat* to include an existential threat to the body-self, the individual self-narration. This scenario relates a story of a patient who sustained a motorcycle accident with significant physical injuries, an event that is assumed to carry the risk of death. After that near-death experience, the patient is left with multiple disruptions in the body, self, and social domains. It is these disruptions which I believe are comparable to Rivers's "existential threat" that initiate the healing ritual.

Dr. Williamson said to Dr. Johnson, "Did you hear about that patient who had a traumatic urethral disruption?"[1] He described the injury in detail. "Dr. Fields got to scrub in. He told me that the patient was riding a motorcycle and he hit a pole, flying forward, striking his groin against something hard, and disrupting the urethra." Dr. Williamson then shrugged his shoulders and made a face as he walked away. Later in the clinic session it became apparent he had not yet seen the patient but he had already heard about the case from the other residents.

Carmen brought the patient back to an exam room. The patient was holding a urine bag out in the open and the wife was walking behind him texting on her phone, looking at the phone and not looking at where she was walking. Carmen took his blood pressure and said, "It is 129/100. That's good."

"I've had a stressful day."

"You're allergic to IVP[2] dye, right?"

"Yeah."

After seeing the patient, Dr. Williamson was standing around the documentation counter, chatting. Dr. Jeffries interrupted and asked, "How far out?"

Dr. Williamson said, "Two weeks. He's comfortable with meds, he's had a bowel movement, he still continues to have perineal[3] swelling."

Dr. Jeffries interrupted saying, "What do you want to do for him?" As they reviewed the chart Dr. Jeffries said, "He's really three weeks out." He then described a butterfly hematoma[4] and indicated that the patient had surgery on July 1, at which point he took his smartphone out and showed the trauma case photos to the residents, "There was significant peritoneal as well as perineal hematoma."[5]

Dr. Williamson said, "So what you want to do?"

Dr. Jeffries replied, "I would do an antegrade and cystoscopy[6] through the suprapubic tube trying to thread a catheter from the bladder through the penis. The tissue during the initial operation was dog meat." He indicated that the catheter would provide a lattice for healing and decrease the possibility of requiring a post-repair urethroplasty.[7] He concluded by saying, "I don't want to do anything. If we do something it will cause increased incontinence, increased impotence. I would only intervene after the first suprapubic catheter change. That's the miracle of embryology: those cells will seek to find each other and essentially close the traumatic laceration naturally."

At that point, we all went into the room. Dr. Jeffries interviewed the patient a little bit. He then asked to examine the patient. Anticipating the emotional response to examining traumatized genitalia, he said, "Don't worry. It's what we do."

After the interview and exam, the patient replied, "I've had multiple previous surgeries under Medicaid. Now I'm self-employed, and for some reason my Medicaid lapsed."

Dr. Jeffries said, "Don't worry. We work for University Hospital. They will have someone assist you with insurance. You won't see one red cent of the bill." Almost imperceptibly, I observed a small tear welling up in the patient's eyes as Dr. Jeffries made this commonplace reassurance.

Dr. Jeffries then asked the patient, "This is a little bit of a personal question, but have you had an erection since the accident?"

The patient said, "Last Thursday I woke up with an erection. It scared the hell out of me. I thought everything was going to explode. I was terrified."

Dr. Jeffries smiled and said, "I've been a urologist for 17 years and nobody died of an erection. The cavernosal artery fills it with blood.[8] Having an erection is a very good sign."

The patient said, "It scared the hell out of me."

Dr. Jeffries asked, "Was it uncomfortable?"

"No."

The conversation then went on to scheduling. Dr. Jeffries said, "I would prefer to do it August 1, giving at least a month before touching anything. I'm going to go out to schedule it."

The wife left the room asking if she could go to the bathroom. Dr. Jeffries was doing other things, but before he could go see the next patient, she pulled him aside and said, "Could I have a minute of your time before you go back in the room? I'm planning to go up north to visit my parents. I go every year. I don't want to go if he is going to have a problem. Also, he's concerned about missing work for financial reasons." She had Dr. Jeffries cornered in an empty exam room for a fairly extensive time and then said, "Give me a few minutes to get back in the room. I don't want him to know that we talked." She then went back into the exam room with her husband.

Dr. Jeffries did return and talk a little bit more about scheduling. Dr. Jeffries brought up the issue of scheduling and said, "There is no rush for surgery. You won't have any more difficulty functioning than you are now, actually less because the two weeks more of healing time." The issue of billing came up again and Dr. Jeffries reassured him again, at which time the patient became tearful.

The wife then introduced the concept of getting back to work, scheduling the exam, and being comfortable going up north during the next procedure. Dr. Jeffries agreed, "That wouldn't be a problem." The patient then left the room and talked to Barbara, the surgical scheduler.

As Dr. Williamson left the room, he was visibly shaken (emotionally), his color was ashen gray, and he was very quiet, which was unusual, as he usually displayed an overall upbeat, positive, helpful demeanor. The silence was notable.

Dr. Jeffries talked to Dr. Williamson about doing the history and physical, "Some of it is on paper. Make sure all the documentation is ready in terms of scheduling operative time. Do you want to see the CT that was done during the recent hospitalization?" While the patient was scheduling the procedure, the residents and Dr. Jeffries reviewed the CT images in detail. Dr. Jeffries said, "I would like to see the coronal views."[9] They looked at everything with particular interest on where the catheter was placed. Dr. Jeffries said multiple times, "It's in the bladder right? It's not in the bowel?" They reviewed the film three times to try to make that determination.

One of the residents asked, "Do you wait six weeks after the injury to do the surgery?"

Dr. Jeffries turned and said, "I personally always wait at least eight to ten weeks."

After negotiating an emotionally charged office visit, Dr. Jeffries goes right back to the CT image to review it again. He is reviewing it with the residents to confirm that his anatomical diagnosis is correct – this has important consequences for therapy and outcome. Also, the reason that such a junior resident (Dr. Fields) was able to scrub in and assist on such a major case was that the patient presented to the emergency room of a nearby hospital. The very nature of an emergency room is to stabilize the patient to prevent death. In this case, re-establishing a basic bodily function, eliminating urine, was an existential threat, because unless that bodily repair was accomplished in the emergency setting, it is probable that the patient would have died. Evidence for this is the surgery and the surgical photos displayed on the smartphone detailing the injuries. Dr. Jeffries referred to the genital area as "dog meat" when he was showing the residents the extent of the injury. The anatomy is not even recognizable to the surgeon and the "repair" required to address the existential threat was to create an alternative urinary system with the suprapubic catheter and urine collection bag that replaced the urethra and bladder during this time of bodily disruption. The intent in this chapter is to establish the initiation to the healing ritual, which I argue is an existential threat. I believe the nature of the clinical case is a good example of the initiation of healing rituals.

I present this scenario to highlight other existential threats to the self, or narrated body-self. Although the patient is not narrating his illness story, he does provide display emotions that are social communications about his experience. Notably, the tears and tearfulness related to the financial disruption of losing Medicaid and not having insurance is a direct threat to initiating and maintaining the healing ritual. Not all doctors are willing to see patients without insurance or even patients with inadequate insurance. The relative importance of this interaction between the patient and Dr. Jeffries was underemphasized in the context of the healing ritual of the office visit, but I attribute this to the narrative structure of healing rituals. Dr. Jeffries simply did not perceive it as important to his job of presiding over the ritual; he would rather look at the CT scan, verify that he placed the catheter anatomically correctly, and plan further medical-surgical management. Imagine this patient telling his friends about his accident and the visit to the doctor – the tearfulness about lost insurance would probably attain greater "Labovian reportability" in such an "illness narrative"; that tearfulness will turn into hundreds of words.

Likewise, there is a discrepancy of perception related to the patient's erection. The patient was "terrified it was going to explode" and said, "It scared the hell out of me," something I claim is a statement of an existential threat (but could also be understood a vestigial illness narrative), while Dr. Jeffries was happy the cavernosal artery was patent or intact. Dr. Williamson was a newlywed with a young infant. Simply observing the "dog meat" of another man's procreative organs after a motor vehicle accident affected him emotionally (his ashen appearance), despite his training to maintain the role of the objective observer. Again, this experience is not enacted as part of the healing ritual and although these experiences by the patient and the resident were observable, they were underemphasized in the structure of the office visit. The existential threat and initiation of the healing ritual structured the office visit.

Through the lens of healing narrative as healing ritual, this scenario highlights the transformative nature of the process. It is a before-and-after situation. Labov might say the first declarative clause was, "The patient had a motor vehicle accident." The second declarative clause was, "The patient's bodily functions were disrupted." I would add that the healing ritual in Western biomedicine is the same as other places and other times – the existential threat of disease (physical trauma) and death brings the patient and the doctor together and initiates the healing ritual.

Patient cognitive models versus doctors' cognitive models

Again, the following brief scenario demonstrates that the patient and the doctor may disagree about the cause of the existential threat, but they both acknowledge one exists. Even that is enough to initiate the healing ritual.

Dr. Stein said to the patient, "We looked at the CT scan. The kidney is this big," he indicated by showing the size with his hands. "We can show you [on the computer screen]." But then he started drawing it and said, "This is the shape of your kidney, and down here there's a solid mass. Usually this is kidney cancer, and the treatment is surgical removal. If there's no spread, you can consider this a cure."

The patient replied, "My husband died four years ago from renal failure, so when you mention 'kidney,' I become uneasy. My primary care physician told me that the lymph nodes were small and that was a good thing because it meant that it probably not spread. I would like it done as soon as possible."

The patient is concerned about death from kidney failure, based on her experience with her husband. There is a high chance she attributes loss of part of her kidney with decreased kidney function – her existential threat. For Dr. Stein, the existential threat would be the spread of the kidney cancer. Although never clarified, the healing ritual proceeded without interruption or clarification. The patient scheduled the surgery.

The patient's explanation of existential threat

This next quotation occurred after one of the patients I interviewed asked me if I had ever had cancer. I told her I had not. Her next words were:

Well then, when you're told that you have cancer, it terrifies you. It surprises you, you're totally confused. You don't know what's going on. So when you meet a doctor who's saying no you're not going to have side effects, no, we caught this early. That gives you reassurance and also makes you look at him like hey, he's going to help me. And that's very important when you see a doctor. I was seeing another doctor who didn't even call to tell me that the results showed I had cancer and that irritated me. I was thinking that this isn't because I have a pimple on my face. This is my life and this is life-threatening.

That last sentence, "This is my life and this is life-threatening," was reason enough to engage in a healing ritual.

In Appendix A of this book, individuals tell their story. Paul describes the liminality provoked by an existential threat and being cut off from society as a difficulty telling his friends he has cancer. Tony describes the existential threat of potentially having cancer as a "mini-breakdown" when the potential of having a life-threatening disease finally hits him, and Alfred worries about the social estrangement in the environment of a retirement community, not so much as death, but as urinary incontinence.

To summarize, it is a threat to the narrating self that forms the existential threat. Narrative disruption or lack of cohesion is about the existence of the narrator and a narrative force – the self. This key concept – existential threat that provokes a type of liminality – as a component of healing rituals was described in the anthropological canon before "healing" took a "narrative turn." It was easy for me to find evidence of such a threat in my data.

Notes

1   The urethra is the tube-like structure in the penis through which urine flows.
2   IVP is an acronym for intravenous pyelogram (dye), a way to improve the x-ray image of the kidney and the urinary collecting system.
3   The anatomical area surrounding the anus, scrotum, and penis.
4   The word "butterfly" describes the shape of the hematoma which resulted from the mechanism of injury.
5   A hematoma is a collection of blood that displaces the tissue and normal anatomy.
6   Direct visualization of the inside of the bladder cavity.
7   Surgical repair of the urethra, the tube through which urine exits the body.
8   This refer to the artery that fills the penis with blood.
9   The coronal view is one of the three axes that planar images of three-dimensional objects can be displayed on the computer.

11 Qualifications of a leech

If Western biomedicine is a healing ritual, then my data should contain observations to verify this. Society confers the privilege of pronouncing a diagnosis narrative only to those who earn the qualifications and credentials (Fortes 1987: 10). Once achieved, others recognize that authority. This training not only qualifies the practitioner to proclaim a diagnosis but the concomitant authority is a vital aspect of the persuasion component of the healing ritual. Although a supportive function, it is a necessary function and intimately connected to the other narrative components of the ritual. It identifies an authoritative narrator.

Transfer of knowledge from teacher to pupil

In the chapter on ritual, I pointed out that there is a transfer of money from student to teacher. Although Rivers was talking about healing rituals in Melanesia, that same statement is a fairly accurate description of post-graduate medical education in the United States. Consider that Dr. Fields has $240,000 of educational debt. In addition to monetary payment, there are many other requirements to "earn" the right to be a healer (Rivers 2001 [1924]: 41; Evans-Pritchard 1976: 97).

The inpatient urology rounding team consists of a chief resident, senior residents, the intern, and finally the medical students. A strict hierarchy is enforced, with the chief resident acting as proxy for the attending physicians for clinical management of the patients, supervising the junior residents. The chief resident also decides who gets to scrub in on what surgery. The chief himself claims the difficult cases and the robotic cases; the others have to wait until they become senior enough or chief to have this opportunity. On the other extreme is the intern who does the repetitive, routine surgical cases, such as retrograde urograms and cystoscopies. In the following vignette, notice how strictly the hierarchy is enforced. The slight infraction is punished by comments about getting experience in the operating room and the ultimate insult to a resident, offering the first assistant position to a medical student.

Connaught Cancer Institute rents renovated floor space on the fifth floor of Hopewell Hospital. The accreditation for the urology residency is through Connaught, so they see most of their patients on this floor. However, they also see consultations on other floors of the interconnected hospitals. Rounds start at 6:30 a.m., so I tried to arrive slightly earlier. The medical students were already there and collecting data from the various computers as well as a perfunctory interview with each patient. Shortly after I arrived, Dr. Wright showed up and immediately went to the computer and started jotting down labs. The tall medical student was doing the identical procedure with a different computer, jotting down labs, both of them copying them onto a computer printout with the patients' names. After Dr. Pinder arrived, he started whispering with Dr. Wright. Shortly thereafter Dr. Wright says, "What do we have here?" The medical student started presenting patient after patient to Dr. Pinder. He reported symptoms, lab results, temperature, and vital signs,[1] including input and output.[2]

At 6:48 a.m., Dr. Fields joined the group. Dr. Pinder said, "Dr. Fields just wants to show up and operate while I take care of patients. At least he wants to go to OR now, so that's a little bit of progress." Rounds continued without comment. Dr. Fields took one of the portable computers on the small tabletop and pushed it around down the hallway and into each individual patient room. He was constantly staring at the computer and typing throughout the walk, the discussion, and the patient interviews. I was able to get a very close look at the computer that Dr. Fields was using. I was able to ascertain that it was actually progress notes that he was generating directly into the computer program.

While in a room with a patient, Dr. Pinder asked, "Are you passing any gas?"

The patient replied, "Why do you say that?" There was no response from Dr. Pinder. Dr. Pinder put gloves on and examined one patient's wound while asking "Any nausea or vomiting?" after finding out the patient had not yet passed gas. Instead, Dr. Pinder started examining the incision and asked, "Any pain?" The only response was "Arrghr-rrghh!" Even while the patient was moaning, Dr. Pinder said, "Incision looks good. We started TPN yesterday."[3]

The patient asked, "Can the drain come out?"

Dr. Pinder said, "Yeah, there's not a lot draining. The incisions look good. Your urine looks good too [even though it was bloody red]. You have a low-grade fever," which seemed to surprise the patient. Dr. Pinder continued, "The most important thing is to use this device," referring to the incentive spirometer. "You should get up and walk around, and perhaps you can get the urinary catheter out today and maybe even possibly go home." As everyone left the room, Dr. Fields pushed the computer on wheels outside the room.

Once we were outside the room and back the hallway, Dr. Fields said to
Dr. Pinder, "This is the first time in my entire residency that I've been
late; it's been 14 months and this is the first time. You showed up two
minutes before I did."
Dr. Pinder said, "It doesn't matter what time I show up."
Dr. Fields replied, "I was hoping you wouldn't chew me out on rounds."
The conversation drifted to "What's the case today?" Then someone
said, "There are four cases tomorrow." Dr. Wright turned toward the
medical students saying, "You might be the first assistant on one of
the surgeries." The entire time the residents were discussing surgeries
and surgical techniques. One of the senior residents used hand gestures in three-dimensional space to demonstrate anatomy and surgical
techniques, another example of using the body to demonstrate three-
dimensional cognitions. He did this multiple times. Once, when they
were arguing about a specific procedure, one of the residents demonstrated a reported technique from the literature and performed the
entire operation in three-dimensional space with his hands to show the
others.

The constant conversation and gesturing about surgical techniques was
always part of the daily discourse in the life of a resident. They are learning their craft – surgical skills. They also have to learn cognitive skills. On
Friday mornings, there is a conference at the residency office attended by a
couple of attending physicians and the residents, followed by an unstructured learning session for residents led by the chief resident. The typical
format for this would be to review board questions from a board exam
preparation book.

The pretense for the meeting was to study. They asked questions from a
textbook. They would intersperse clinical case discussions with test questions and socializing:

In contrast to the admiration and banter with their own faculty, they discussed the strengths and weaknesses of private attending physicians
with an almost mocking perspective. They said things like, "He went
crazy on me" or "That was when I was the most uncomfortable, when
we went in to see a guy dying from cancer and [this particular attending
physician] said, 'Hey you're dying of cancer. How's life, huh, big guy?' "
or "He's the best one to be on call with. He's an Iron Curtain."
They were also joking about the attending, and one of the residents had asked
a particular community attending, "How do you do a hydrocoele?"[4]
The attending replied, "I open the scrotum. I take it out." The resident was
aghast that he didn't have any particular procedure and was unfamiliar
with a particular named procedure that Dr. Patel uses. When the resident questioned the community attending, he reportedly said, "I don't
know what you're talking about."

In addition to sharing surgical techniques and medical management knowledge, the topic discussed the most was the amount of surgical experience
each of them had, and how they could get more experience. A junior
resident said, "I beat him by an hour [arriving at the hospital], so I did
the surgery and I was actually leaving by the time the senior resident
got there." Another resident pointed out, "The next senior should get
there late, because I want a chance to have opportunities [to do such
big surgery] myself."

Another resident said, "I saw an autotransplant. It was a sweet case. It failed
miserably." This willingness to gain experience without benefit to the
patient was echoed by another resident's comment, "We have to do a
stat prostatectomy before they diagnose the lung cancer."[5] The residents
talked about a retroperitoneal varicocele[6] repair and the senior residents
said, "What's the plan for that case? I plan on scrubbing, but if one of
you guys wanted to do it, I'll walk you through it."

"He let you do one of those?"

The senior resident said, "Those guys [at an affiliated hospital] are open
surgeons, so they are more comfortable letting you do things that are
open, because they know that they can get you out of trouble. They are
less comfortable letting us use the robot. That's totally different with Dr.
Jeffries." They talked about the different robotic surgeries each resident
had done and the senior resident said, "The Cowboys are in town, and
that's never going to happen again." He was referring to the episode
where one of the junior residents did more robotic surgeries than one of
the senior residents. "That was selfish of them. You're still third in line.
Just remember that."

This desire for surgical experience is understandable. It is the only way to
achieve competence. On a different occasion, I overheard Dr. Jeffries telling the residents that he would be happy to confront the private attending
physicians if they were not allowing the residents to get enough experience. Because robotic surgery is relatively new, patients seek experienced
surgeons. This measure of experience both creates the hierarchy and the
hierarchy ensures that each resident is trained properly. Consider the socialization process of the more junior residents:

Dr. Fields was one of the least experienced residents, still in his first year.
During the morning "education" session described earlier, the conversation drifted to a clinical discussion of the patient who had a PSA of 10.6
without any rectal manipulation. He said there were some pulmonary
findings. Someone asked Dr. Fields, "How big was the prostate?"

He replied, "It was hard to feel. This is a problem: how are you supposed to
know how big it is, because there is no frame of reference?"

Another resident said, "People want a number. Just do the exam and then
guesstimate."

Dr. Fields mentioned, "After the beginning of the New Year, there will be
a general surgery resident on the urology service, and then there will
finally be someone lower on the totem pole than me. I'm looking forward to them carrying the pager because it's very annoying trying to
answer the pager while being scrubbed in and answering questions
through the nurse. I had to do two internships, one general surgery
internship and one urology internship, and during both I'm the lowest
person on the totem pole."

As if to add insult to injury, Dr. Fields said, "I have $240,000 in educational
debt. I lost my deferment, so now they take the money right out of my
debit account every month."

Dr. Solski walked over to Dr. Fields and slapped him on the back hugging
his shoulders, reassuring him it will be okay.

This is validation of the apprentice role in the healing ritual described by
Rivers in the chapter on ritual. Not only do senior residents teach junior
residents; attending doctors teach residents.

Although I wrote mostly about the role of how doctors interact with
patients, I would be remiss if I did not describe the obvious affection the
attending physicians had for the residents and vice versa. Additionally,
although the residents have to negotiate a difficult hierarchy, they looked
out for each other, as evidenced by Dr. Solski giving Dr. Fields a hug of
encouragement. In fact, the group recognized the stress Dr. Fields was experiencing; they decided to "skip school," and the entire group decided to
go to the Farmer's Market. Everyone drove separately, so Dr. Fields told
me I could ride with him. (I was even lower in the hierarchy, as I described
earlier.) His car was an older model and obviously needed repair. During the
ride, he continued to talk about how difficult the training experience was.
When we arrived, the group decided to go to a candy store – literally, it was
like kids in a candy store, despite the fact that these were grown men. It
was impossible not to appreciate the affection and caring they had for each
other. They cheered up Dr. Fields using playful goofing off behaviors and
telling crude jokes. They talked about relationships at home, starting a family, aspirations for their future, but mostly about how to survive. They were
all enduring this liminal coming of age apprenticeship together. I could not
help but think this was a ritual within a ritual. Their training carried a huge
personal sacrifice for each of them. After this "morning off work" interlude,
they had to return to work.

Consider the following Socratic teaching interactions during inpatient
oncology rounds:

Dr. Spangler asked, "Why doesn't he sleep?"
One resident answered, "He told me because of his headache."
Another resident said, "Because he's restless."

Dr. Spangler said, "It's not because he's having a heart attack, is it?" At that point, they listed all the different causes of mental status change, including infection, myocardial infarction,[7] stroke, etc.

One of the residents said, "We didn't get an MRI."

Then Dr. Spangler said, "What else?"

The presenting resident suggested, "Psychiatry problems or medication."

Dr. Spangler said, "What would give you mental status changes with gait changes?"

"Normal pressure hydrocephalus."[8]

Then Dr. Spangler said, "What else?"

The resident guessed, "HIV."

Dr. Spangler said, "No!" quite emphatically and repeated "No!" slapping the table. "What about a sleeper?" (She was referring to a hypnotic medicine.) "We need to think about it like a good internist."

The resident said, "He seems a little odd [referring to the patient]."

Dr. Spangler then interrupted and went back to her previous line of thought, "We missing one more. There's one more." There was relative silence, and Dr. Spangler continued, "I must've tortured you at least once this month about this." None of the residents could come up with the answer, and so Dr. Spangler told them "Thyroid problems." Her conclusion on this case was, "We don't know what's going on. Let's wait for the scan."

Dr. Spangler was doing some more teaching, "Where does lung cancer metastasize to? It's a really tiny gland."

The presenting residents guessed, "The pituitary."

Dr. Spangler laughed, bending down and putting her forehead on the table while laughing. When she rose back up, Dr. Spangler said, "The gland I'm looking for is close to the liver." The post call resident couldn't figure it out and finally Dr. Spangler said, "It's the adrenal gland."

In a deadpan voice, the post call resident replied, "Which is also close to the liver." This joke was irony because the pituitary is in the skull and not at all close to liver.

Dr. Spangler used this teaching technique a lot. This next section demonstrates the relationship of a CT scan to nausea, followed by teaching about causes of nausea:

The next patient was a transferred from Benedict Hospital. There was no notification to the resident prior to the patient arriving on the floor, to which Dr. Spangler expressed her displeasure. The patient had just gotten his first dose of cisplatin[9] and he started vomiting, so his mom called and took him back to the hospital. In the emergency room at Benedict Hospital, they did an x-ray and a CT scan determining there was no obstruction, so he was sent back to Connaught. The discussion continued about multiple reasons why they couldn't start chemotherapy.

Dr. Atlas went to the computer and looked at the CT scan. Dr. Spangler replied, "He never had puke problems before," and then went over four different reasons for nausea. "The first one is anticipatory nausea. That's when the patient is approaching the chemotherapy suite and starts to get nauseated. That's the right answer on the test. The second type is acute nausea. That's with the initiation of the chemotherapy right at the moment of chemotherapy infusion. Chemotherapy-related nausea, which is the third type, which is after the patient's had the treatment."

Dr. Atlas piped in, "Non-chemo-related nausea."

Dr. Spangler asked, "What's the next kind?" Nobody could provide an answer. "The fourth type is chronic nausea, which means it's there all the time despite chemo or the disease. No one can find the reason."

This type of Socratic teaching occurred in all types of settings whenever doctors of different hierarchical status worked together. At one point, the emeritus urology professor, Dr. Bridges, was supervising an operating room case when Dr. Stein stopped by to watch Dr. Wright and Dr. Fields perform a retrograde uroscopy and cystoscopy with biopsy. Dr. Stein asked a trick question about how to locate the source of malignant cells in a complex clinical situation. They all discussed the case. Even the medical student joined in the mind-teaser, and despite the input of the chief resident, the senior resident, and all the others, no one could figure out the answer to the question. This type of cognitive practice occurred abstractly or related to the clinical case at the time. I have described these social practices for achieving competence elsewhere (Meza and Provenzano 2015).

In addition to all the learning described earlier, residents reviewed CT scans and MRI images as part of daily activities. Whenever a resident was in clinic, the attending physician always reviewed the images with the resident. During each of these encounters, the resident always reviewed the images together with the attending physician during the clinical encounter as part of the apprenticeship of becoming competent. Learning the "ways of the occult" establish induction into the ways of the healer. Residents reviewed images in clinic, at Multidisciplinary Care Conference, in the operating room, and on rounds in the hospital. Residents reviewed images as often as attending physicians, which was practically on every case.

The healing ritual is a cultural production, and in order for it to survive, there must be cultural replication. This is partly accomplished through the specialized training required to perform healing rituals. Without this specialized knowledge, the ritual would not be effective. In multiple settings during fieldwork, I observed residents working closely with senior faculty, reviewing computer images, answering Socratic questions, and practicing motor skills in the hallways and in the operating room. The residents "pay" for the specialized healing skills that create the expertise to claim socially recognized power by long work hours, studying, apprenticeship-like workdays, and the all-important surgical experience. This learning process is all implicit. At no time were the "qualifications of a leech" described overtly as learning how to make a diagnosis narrative or even the more remote concept of healing. These last two concepts are anthropological insights that arise from observing daily routines.

Notes

1 Vital signs include blood pressure, pulse or heart rate, temperature, respiratory or breathing rate, and "pain."
2 Measures of fluids going into the body and fluids coming out of the body, recorded in the nursing notes section of the chart.
3 TPN is an acronym for total parenteral nutrition – all nutrition provided through an IV and not the gastrointestinal system.
4 A hydrocoele is a cyst on the spermatic cord; when very large it can cause discomfort, the reason to surgically remove it.
5 Stat, or STAT, refers to immediate; prostatectomy is surgical removal of the prostate gland. In this case, the residents were joking about how to get more surgical experience. If lung cancer was diagnosed, the patient would not be eligible for a prostatectomy.
6 Retroperitoneal refers to anatomical structures behind ("retro") the abdominal cavity, which is covered with a membrane called the peritoneum. Varicocele refers to "varicose veins" or engorged veins in the scrotum.
7 Heart attack.
8 This type of social interaction in medical education is called "pimping" after a famous article in *JAMA* in 1980. She is asking them what she is thinking as a method for them to recognize diseases, syndromes, or diagnoses.
9 A toxic cancer chemotherapeutic drug.

References

Fortes, M. 1987. *Religion, Morality, and the Person: Essays on Tallensi Religion*, Cambridge: Cambridge University Press.
Meza, J. P., and A. Provenzano. 2015. Power, Competence, and Professionalism in Medical Education. *MedEdPublish* 5.
Pritchard, E.E.E. 1976. *Witchcraft, Oracles, and Magic Among the Azande*. Oxford: Clarendon Press.
Rivers, W. 2001 [1924]. *Medicine, Magic, and Religion*. London: Routledge Classics.

12 Healing relationships

My data are uniformly consistent in documenting that doctors do not explore the illness experience as part of a routine clinical encounter, yet I observed ample evidence of healing relationships between doctors and patients. The healing ritual facilitates a healing relationship, and the healing relationship generates intimacy that subsequently allows doctors to explore and become part of the patients' experiences, including illness experiences. I suggest that the ill person experiences an existential threat to life, and that is what biomedicine addresses in a very culturally defined way. Sequence matters. Biomedicine and healing relationships are not mutually exclusive, as portrayed by many anthropologists. *I argue that healing relationships result from completion of the healing ritual.*

Authentic relationships between patients and doctors exemplify the classic definition of healing relationships as "knowing the whole person." I present observations that indicate such relationships are commonplace in the context of a biomedical clinical encounter.

Some anthropologists portray Western biomedicine as devoid of meaningful interpersonal relationships between doctors and patients. Yet I observed the opposite: patients loved their doctors. My first clue as to how this attachment formed occurred on inpatient rounds with Dr. Smith:

I arrived at Connaught inpatient unit early, approximately 6:15 in the morning. Dr. Williamson walked in and looked somewhat non-communicative, not smiling, and there was no specific greeting for me. Shortly after that, Dr. Johnson walked in, and they were side by side on computers both retrieving lab work in preparation for rounds. Dr. Smith showed up while Dr. Johnson and Dr. Williamson were still working, looking up labs and x-rays. There were apparently only three patients on the service and Dr. Williamson said, "One of them should go home. He looks pretty good numbers-wise."
While still in front of the computers, reviewing an abdominal x-ray, Dr. Smith said, "Who is it we consulted for G.I.?[1] I forget – it's been so long. Maybe we should think about a cardiologist."
Dr. Johnson said, "It's just sinus tachy.[2] It's probably not his heart. We just have an ECG."[3]

"I like to rule everything out," Dr. Smith replied.

The first patient we saw engaged in an extensive negotiation about an NG tube. The patient said, "It causes severe pain, and I want it out as soon as possible." The residents had previously looked at this x-ray when they were making sit-down rounds in front of the computers. He had multiple air fluid levels[4] since surgery (which is why they had consulted gastroenterology). Dr. Smith acknowledged his perspective, acknowledged his pain, and explained why it was necessary to keep the NG tube in, telling him they would check later.[5]

The patient questioned, "How much later?"

"We'll check back later in the day."

"I can't wait until you finished in the operating room."

Both Dr. Smith and Dr. Johnson asked his cooperation and finally they came to a compromise solution, "If you leave it in a couple more hours we could have the nurse page us."

The next patient was talkative and comfortable. Dr. Smith said, "You did well." In this case, Dr. Smith did most of the interacting with the patient. I had the sense that there was a natural rapport between the two of them, more than typical for a resident physician.

Dr. Smith asked him, "How did this all start?"

The patient said, "Ten days ago there wasn't anything wrong with me, this was simply something they found. I heard of Connaught, and that's why I came here." The patient had a large, well-healed nephrectomy scar but had severe tape burns with open ulcerations.

Dr. Smith examined him and said, "No more silk tape for him [to the other residents] . . . Is the Norco[6] helping with the pain? [to the patient]."

The patient asked about his prescription for narcotics when he went home. "Right now I need it every four hours, because if it goes to the fifth hour it starts hurting severely. When it heals, I won't need it anymore, and I'll cut back."

While leaving the room, Dr. Smith said, "I cannot argue with you because you carry a gun." After getting out of the room Dr. Smith said, "The security officer came up to visit the patient and told me to take good care of him because the patient was a police officer."

When dictating the field notes of those interactions, I noticed that the conversation was a lot more personal than typical for morning rounds. I couldn't help but think that Dr. Smith had been the resident to operate on the policeman.

The next day, I asked Dr. Smith if that was true and he said, "Yes." I had written in my scratch notes next to Dr. Smith's name: "tender caring bedside manner." I showed him what I had written and he replied, "That extra 30 seconds to a minute makes a big difference, even if you just listen. Sometimes it works, and sometimes it doesn't. You can tell the patients like it. Like the patient with the small bowel obstruction.

Sometimes I go up there in the afternoon when I have nothing to do and spend five minutes just talking, but not necessarily about his medical condition. I think it helps the patient to talk to the doctor about things other than what's going on; otherwise, you don't know anything about him and nothing about the context of the patient's illness. I think it makes it better." He then indicated that he had done the surgery for the patient with the bowel obstruction and NG tube as well. I told him how impressed I was about what he said, and he continued, "If you don't do that stuff, you're just wasting your time. Anybody can learn the science."

The next day, Dr. Smith emailed me his personal statement that he was submitting for his fellowship applications. Although it was personal, he wrote about the same topic of knowing the patient intimately. This was very revealing data.

Dr. Smith actually used the word "illness," one of the only times I heard the word used during my entire fieldwork. He contrasted "science" and "knowing about the patient." His caring bedside manner was everything patients could wish for as a compassionate physician caring for patients. The important observation was that these behaviors occurred only with the patients he personally operated on and only *after* he had operated on them. This episode caused me to re-evaluate all of my data, searching to see if this pattern was consistent. Going through my field notes, I was able to confirm this pattern. In all sites and for each doctor, with patients being evaluated for surgery or treatment, there was a respect and attentiveness to the patient and the patient's needs. For follow-up visits after therapy, there was laughter, fondness, open displays of affection, and a different level of sharing, often on a personal level, which was totally absent prior to surgery or therapy.

I recorded a clinical encounter in the outpatient clinic when Dr. Jeffries was running almost two hours behind schedule. None of the patients complained or showed any irritation when he finally entered the exam room. For one patient, the visit was a routine follow-up. Dr. Jeffries merely ordered trivial labs during a very brief visit. When Dr. Jeffries apologized for the long wait, the patient said, "It's no problem. I gave up three previous urologists for you. For you I would do anything." This statement by the patient demonstrates an allegiance and tolerance beyond what could be expected without a healing relationship. As we were leaving the exam room, Dr. Jeffries told me that he had resected a renal cancer for her nine years ago. Again, in a manner similar to Dr. Smith, there was an understanding and healing relationship forged by surviving the existential threat together as a doctor-patient team. The doctor is allowed to enter the liminal social space of disease and it is the shared experiences that creates the interpersonal relationship of intimacy, a form of *communitas*. Enacting a healing ritual (resection of the kidney cancer) allowed me to observe a different type of the interpersonal relationship between the doctor and the patient.

The same is true for Dr. Stein:

Dr. Stein said, "Every single year Rabbi Levine sends me a message on Rosh
Hashanah. Rosh Hashanah begins tonight and is a time when you're
supposed to contemplate life, what your life is all about, the fact that
you're alive and not dead. Rabbi Levine sends me a thank-you note
every year for being alive because I performed his surgery. He's still
alive. There were all these men with black hats and black coats [Dr.
Stein took his hand and made swirling motions of the side of his face
indicating the Hasidic curls]. At the time of the surgery, he had people
praying at the Western Wall to guide my hands during surgery. In his
annual thank-you note he mentions that he's thankful that my hands
performed the surgery well."

Both Dr. Jeffries's patient and Dr. Stein's story confirm what I learned from
Dr. Smith. I noticed a change in the doctor-patient relationship before the
diagnosis and treatment compared to after the diagnosis and treatment.
I concluded that the intimacy and personal knowledge of the "whole person" by the doctor is a consequence of the healing ritual, not a prerequisite;
healing relationships are authentic relationships where there is no barrier to
sharing between the patient and the doctor.

There are multiple other examples. The urologists were not treating a
decontextualized "body organ," as described in the anthropological canon.
During office visits with patients, while simply following up for cancer surveillance (post-surgical), Dr. Jeffries talked with his patients about all types
of social aspects of their life. He talked about NASCAR with his patient
who was a NASCAR fan; he talked about local politics with his patient who
habitually wrote letters to the editor of a small-town newspaper; he knew
all the patients' family members and asked about them when they didn't
show up. He listened to their concerns about money, their travel plans,
their worries, and their hopes for the future. He advocated and guided them
about how to manipulate the healthcare system to get catheters or dressing
changes, and so forth. When a patient talked about getting readmitted to the
hospital, Dr. Jeffries joked, "You should get in-store credit – every seventh
admission is free." When patients complained about hospital food or bad
coffee, he replied, "That's how they plan to get people out of the hospital."
The patients also knew details of his personal life. When asked what type
of car he drove, Dr. Jeffries was quick to respond: "An F150." Dr. Jeffries
also shared information about his vacations and the school activities of his
children. These are intimate details demonstrating the depth of trust embedded in these relationships.

After this point in the fieldwork, I started to look more closely to verify
this finding because it was the exact opposite of my preconceptions of the
temporal sequence of healing relationships based on Kleinman's model.
After reviewing all of my data, there was not a single episode of this type of
banter and intimacy during the formulation of a diagnostic narrative and

treatment plan. Those visits were always respectful and attentive in a polite way, but there was no sharing of any personal information as I describe earlier. Sharing personal information with patients is a form of intimacy, a hallmark of a healing relationship. Self-disclosure is just that: a narrating self disclosing information about the self. The act of disclosing is evidence of a self recognizing the other as a like being with a mental life similar to one's own. The turning point or transformation in the doctor-patient relationship, with regard to intimacy, candor, and allegiance, was always after the completion of the ritual of diagnosis and treatment. I believe that the existential threat alienates a patient from normal social status and function and that through the shared journey through that liminality into a transformed social space, forms the bond of the authentic doctor-patient relationship. It reminds me of the brotherhood forged among combat units in the military. I suggest these examples demonstrate that a transformation occurs in the doctor-patient relationship that results in the doctor knowing "the whole person," the definition of an authentic relationship. Hence, the illness narrative is not missing or ignored by biomedical practitioners; in fact, it is the exact opposite. Anthropologists simply looked in the wrong places based on preconceived notions of healing.

Perhaps the best data, and certainly the most convincing observations to verify this assertion regarding the transformation of the doctor-patient relationship, occurred with Dr. Spangler. I observed her on inpatient oncology rounds prior to observing her in the outpatient clinic. She was not the attending physician of record for the patients in the hospital. She was merely supervising their care when they were in the hospital. The vast majority of the time at the inpatient site she spent teaching and reviewing cases, hardly spending any time at all in the room with the patients. The few minutes she did spend with them, her demeanor was cut-and-dried, merely informing them of management decisions that had already been made when discussing their cases earlier. This was consistent over the approximately forty patients I observed on the inpatient service.

In contrast, for patients that she saw in the outpatient clinic, she was the attending physician and directly participated in the oncology diagnosis and oncology treatment plan. Her behavior was instantly changed. In the outpatient clinic, she hugged nearly every patient, greeted them with enthusiasm, teased them about their foibles, fussed over their difficulties. Her naturally bubbly personality was openly displayed with the patients and they reciprocated. She knew the life story of every patient. Again, these patients had experienced the existential threat of the healing ritual together with her, the authentic relationships where total honesty and open discussions about things medical and things meaningful were on full display.

We then went back into the room and Dr. Spangler gave the patient a large hug.

The patient asked, "Could I have a B12 shot for energy?"

Dr. Spangler said, "Sure," and then told Dr. Atlas to make arrangements for it.

Dr. Atlas appeared uncomfortable and then told the patient, "You are taking all kinds of supplements for energy and you don't need B12 because you're taking a multiple vitamin tablet that has B12 in it."

Dr. Spangler told the patient, "You can have it," and then Dr. Spangler started teasing Dr. Atlas in the exam room. Dr. Spangler self-disclosed that she herself was vitamin D deficient.

Eventually Dr. Atlas said, "I don't think a B12 shot is necessary."

Dr. Spangler told the patient, "It's his fault." Continuing, she asked, "Did the radiation oncologist do a rectal exam?"

The patient said, "Yep, and I asked him if he should have both hands on my shoulders during the rectal exam." This comment was ignored.

The conversation drifted to the initial treating urologist at a community hospital and the patient said, "If I saw that guy in the parking lot I would run him over." The office visit concluded, and Dr. Spangler left after giving the patient a hug and then went immediately to her computer.

This interaction is typical. It began with Dr. Spangler hugging her patient, and ended with Dr. Spangler hugging her patient. During the interview, she indulged his request for a B12 shot knowing that it was purely for placebo reasons; the less experienced Dr. Atlas, who didn't have a healing relationship with the patient, wasn't as comfortable. Dr. Spangler tolerated the patient's off-color joke, despite the gender difference between the two of them. Similar to Dr. Jeffries and his patients, Dr. Spangler was perfectly comfortable disclosing her personal health information, that she is vitamin D deficient. This speaks to a level of intimacy and comfort that is remarkable.

The before-and-after aspect of these observations was very apparent when Dr. Spangler was seeing a patient or family for a second opinion. In those instances, she focused purely on the diagnosis narrative. It would be totally inappropriate for her to hug such a patient. I believe this is explained again by the change in relationship that occurs by completing the healing ritual.

Kleinman characterizes the medical record:

> I will first provide a transcript of a doctor-patient interview and then describe the wording of the physician's formal write-up in the patient's record. I don't contend that the following example is representative; indeed I believe that the degree of professional insensitivity it depicts is unusual.
>
> (1988: 131)

The following observation indicates how Kleinman misinterpreted that data:

Dr. Spangler uses a lot of banter with the patients, a lot of joking. She seems to know the life story of each patient extremely well. When she was dictating it was almost a Dr. Jekyll and Mr. Hyde phenomenon because she reverted to strict biomedical language with history and physical formatting. The juxtaposition of the two styles was dramatic. Verbally she said the patient was just a "worry wart" about his sinuses. The patient said that he ordered his own CT scan. Dr. Spangler diagnosed postnasal drip, told him to use saline nasal spray and to not worry about it. When she was dictating the progress note, she said she examined the sinus, there were no lymph nodes, reading all the available labs, and it was the biomedical version of a viral illness and sinus problems.[7] Dr. Spangler is usually very effervescent, poignant, joking with the patients, but when she's dictating she uses a rapid monotone devoid of emotion, a stark contrast to the experience I just observed in the exam room.

As with every other clinical encounter I observed – at the urology clinic, the oncology clinic, or the radiation oncology clinic – the healing relationship in the exam room was never recorded in the medical record. It is an analytic error to conclude that the personal relationship of knowing the patient as a whole person is absent because there is no documentation of it in the medical record. The purpose of the medical record is to record the diagnosis narrative – not reflect the healing relationship.

Kleinman's model begins with empathetic understanding. My observations demonstrated empathetic understanding occurs after completion of the healing ritual:

> We then returned to Dr. Spangler's cubicle. Dr. Spangler said, "I got that email. It was so sad. I called to tell him about his metastatic brain disease. There were three mets on CT of the brain, and I thought I heard the patient crying on the phone. He was actually devastated because his business was bankrupt because an employee of 30 years had embezzled everything. He declined evaluation. The embezzler took everything."

Was this patient quietly crying about the end of his life's work resulting from the betrayal or the end of his life from yet another existential threat? Or both? The doctor was empathetic enough to appreciate the sadness. Dr. Spangler utilized those healing relationships as therapeutic maneuvers:

> I was following Dr. Spangler into the next room and she said to the patient, "We're going to stick together for a good long time. You can't get rid of me. Do you want to start today?"
> He said, "Next office visit."
> She said, "That's what you said last time. It's been two years since you've had it, but you steadfastly refuse." The entire office visit was essentially banter. Dr. Spangler asked, "How's your friend?"
> The patient said, "He is avoiding you. He actually brought me to clinic today."

The friend was also a patient of Dr. Spangler's but he failed to follow up. She said, "Come on, I need to go hassle him," and the patient went out into the lobby. Dr. Spangler followed him and I followed Dr. Spangler. We went out through the doors, and Dr. Spangler walked right into the lobby and sat down next to the gentleman. There were probably 35 people in the waiting room, and she was out there talking to the patient, "You need to follow up."

Dr. Spangler then told me, "I needed to track them down. They're both drinkers."

There is a difference between Dr. Atlas, who hasn't gone through the healing ritual with any of the patients, and Dr. Spangler, who has:

I went with Dr. Atlas to see the next patient. Dr. Atlas said, "You are going to have to decide whether or not you are going to accept treatment, or no treatment, because the chemotherapy you are currently on isn't working. Your PSA level is rising."

The patient said, "My great-grandson is three years old, and he announced to everybody that somebody's going to die and then I won't see them anymore. Two days later my son-in-law in Kansas died of heart problems."

Dr. Atlas went over all of his history of chemotherapy including the entire documentation of the recent rise in the PSA. He did then say, "There are good new experimental drugs that can treat your cancer despite the treatment failure of the current chemotherapy, and so good therapy is still available."

"I've never had any symptoms at all despite my obviously very long history being treated for prostate cancer."

Dr. Spangler went into the room and the patient repeated the entire story to Dr. Spangler. Dr. Spangler hugged the patient on the way in and hugged the patient on the way out again. She did say to the patient, "I am considering no treatment, but I don't want the prostate cancer to get away from us. There's really good treatment. As soon as I get my hands on it, it will be available for you, but in the meantime, I want to go ahead with the experimental protocol." Multiple times when she was in the exam room, the patient referred to records from a different doctor, and she kept turning to say, "We need to get those records. . . . We need to get those records." Dr. Spangler did seem to provide more empathetic statement saying, "I'm sorry for your loss," referring to his son-in-law.

In this example, Dr. Atlas performed a history and physical. The physical exam requires touching the patient in very stylized ways, considered acceptable only in the setting of going to the doctor. This type of touching occurs between strangers in the doctor's office. Dr. Atlas had never met the patient before. Contrast Dr. Atlas's stylized physical exam (the same style Dr. Spangler used at the inpatient setting when she didn't personally know the patients) with Dr. Spangler's abundant use of hugging between herself and patients she treated personally. I contend that "hugging" is a marker for the healing relationship, something that only occurs after performing the healing ritual. In fact, later in my data collection, I was able to discern other doctors say such tender things that I referred to them as "hug equivalents," comparing them to Dr. Spangler's style. Dr. Spangler was able to treat the threat of the son-in-law's death because of her healing relationship with the patient. The contrast between Dr. Atlas and Dr. Spangler in responding to the news of the death in the family was very different. I do not think it was a coincidence: empathy and condolences are socially acceptable. I believe the ability to incorporate it into the clinical encounter is facilitated by having a healing relationship.

Sometimes the healing ritual is cyclical, as with patients who have chronic disease. Consider the following case:

Amber told me the next patient had a PSA of 6,000 and was very weak. He tried to go to one of his children's graduations, but he wasn't able to make it.

Dr. Spangler came in and said the patient whose PSA was 6,000 wasn't taking any pain medicines. "I am going to force him to be treated today because if I let him go he won't come back. I took a look and he's two liters behind." I followed her into the room. His family member was there and Dr. Spangler said emphatically, "You're weak, you're tired, you're getting it treated with chemotherapy." The family member was nodding agreement. Although silent throughout the entire time, the patient was extremely weak. He could barely lift his arm. He was brought in in a transportation chair. Dr. Spangler looked in his mouth; he did appear to be dehydrated. Dr. Spangler then said, "It's a good thing I know you well; I can yell at you." After we left the room, she said she had known him for four years. She had initially met him when he had spinal cord compression and he was severely ill. "When he gets better, he will become noncompliant, and then he comes back when he gets into trouble."

Knowing the patient well enough to be able to yell at them for their own good is a marker of the quality of the relationship.

Healing relationships are authentic relationships. They enable each person to express their full humanity, free of cultural performance, allowing the patient's self to interact directly with the doctor's self in a setting of trust and intimacy. These examples demonstrate that doctor and patient have close intimate, caring relationships – a stark contrast to the caricatured version of biomedicine as an oppressive colonization described by theorists of narrative healing. I discuss the anthropological canon on narrative healing later and offer these relationships I witnessed and write about to counter the "dehumanizing rhetoric of medical anthropologists that strip Drs. Stein, Jeffries, Spangler, and Williamson, etc. of their humanity."

Of particular interest to me is how healing rituals allow the formation of healing relationships. I contend that the healing relationship is the important outcome, a form of *communitas* achieved after traveling through the liminal social space of disease and death. The healing relationship is a moral relationship (Beach and Inui 2006). Viewed in this light, a healing relationship is a refutation of the repeated and forceful critique of biomedicine as inattentive to the illness narrative. Throughout my entire theoretical survey of the anthropological literature, the term healing relationship does not appear. The closest approximations are Kleinman's "medical psychotherapy" and Mattingly's "therapeutic emplotments" and "therapeutic interactions." There is much about "social actors," but that references the person, not the self. It is the relationship of one individual self to another self, as like beings, that forms an authentic relationship (using Kleinman's term). This authentic relationship is the ultimate defense against alienation and, as Tomasello would phrase it, the foundation of culture. I argue that healing rituals foster healing relationships through an experience that has both an antecedent narrative structure and results in an emergent healing narrative.

Notes

1   GI is an acronym for gastrointestinal, or gastroenterology, a medical specialty dealing with the digestive system.
2   Fast heartbeat.
3   ECG is an acronym for electrocardiogram, a tracing of the electrical activity in the heart as measured by transducers placed at specific locations on the skin of the chest.
4   A finding on x-ray indicating the bowels weren't working; there is no propulsion downstream.
5   NG tube, or nasogastric tube, placed through the nose and inserted into the stomach; an extremely noxious procedure when left in any length of time.
6   A brand name of narcotic pain medication.
7   Dr. Spangler wrote the note in a way that precluded recurrent cancer as an explanation for the sinus symptoms.

References

Beach, Mary Catherine, and Thomas Inui. 2006. Relationship-Centered Care – A Constructive Reframing. *Journal of General Internal Medicine* 21(S1):S3–S8.
Kleinman, Arthur. 1988. *The Illness Narratives – Suffering, Healing, and the Human Condition*. New York: Basic Books.

13 When the healing ritual fails

I observed hundreds of office visits, watched many surgeries, attended many conferences and teaching sessions and participated in rounds in the hospital. I base my comments about the diagnosis narrative and healing ritual on those observations. My findings were remarkably consistent across all aspects of my fieldwork. Anthropologists also explore the exception to the rule and learn from those observations as well. I find it remarkable that I found only two office visits that did not fit the pattern I described. Both are presented here; note that both of these examples, the ritual structure was degraded.

In order for a ritual to be efficacious, the leech must be performing the ritual correctly. Any deviation is a cause for failure. Cheryl Mattingly recognized this fact. In one of her more powerful statements, Mattingly says, "Rather than seeing occupational therapy as an 'applied science,' it is perhaps better understood as a kind of healing ritual. . . . Like other healing rituals, therapeutic success depends on the kind of efficacious performance" (Mattingly 1998: 161). From a theoretical perspective, I wholeheartedly concur and this chapter is presented with that statement in mind.

In this chapter, I describe one clinical encounter, a case report in the published anthropological literature, and a second clinical encounter. The first example describes a conflict between an illness narrative and the diagnosis narrative highlighting the failure of the healing ritual when an illness narrative asserts priority.

In the following vignette, the illness narrative disrupts the healing ritual by preventing the doctor in proclaiming a diagnosis. Although the vignette is somewhat long, it is important to count the number of diagnoses offered and the rebuttal by the patient for each diagnosis. There is no agreement to a mutual cultural myth. The patient is "self-diagnosing" with some regularity.

Dr. Jeffries described the patient to me as a real problem and said, "The patient came for a second opinion after being treated at State University for many years. The patient is a 54-year-old woman with scoliosis and multiple urologic surgeries. She is a Jehovah's Witness, and that could be a problem. She's had recurrent urinary tract infections, complaining of incontinence around the stoma as well. She has previously had a bladder augmentation and a sling for the incontinence and eventually wound up with a right hydronephrosis requiring removal of the kidney. She had an ileal loop and her BMI was greater than 40 [morbidly obese]. She has multiple chronic medical problems including restrictive lung disease requiring oxygen at home, coronary artery disease, COPD, and she is coming to me for a third opinion. The last time I met her I had a 'two-hour cyclical conversation.' She brought up her urologic problems, and I explained all of that to her. She brought up her bacterial problems, and I explained all that to her. She brought up multiple other problems, and I explained all that, too. At the end of it I felt bad because for every single other patient the rest of the day I had to apologize because I was so late. After all this discussion, the patient refused ultrasound, refused any blood draw, but did agree to go for urodynamic study, which she had downtown. That did not demonstrate any leaking which was inconsistent with her story. The only surgery would be an ileovesicostomy, but again I'm very concerned about the surgical risk."

Dr. Jeffries told me, "You will see how painful this patient is." Carmen had been trying to put this patient in the room for 25 minutes, and I could overhear the patient talking incessantly. Dr. Jeffries characterized it as cartoon characters where the two of them are fighting and there's a whirlwind and other people get sucked into it. We were sitting there waiting over thirty minutes prior to going to see this patient.

I asked Dr. Jeffries about one of the statements when he said he wanted to help the patient and he replied, "I do want to help her, but I don't want her to die on the [surgical] table. I can't get her to change any of her medicines." He then went on to say, "It's not going to be pleasant." He said, "I'm going to try to put the patient at ease."

Dr. Jeffries said, "I want to see the look on Carmen's face when she walks out of that room."

Indeed Carmen contracted all her facial muscles as she turned the corner when she finally got out of the room. She muttered under her breath, "For the love of God." She then walked over to Dr. Jeffries, gave him a back rub, put her elbow on the charting table, and pushed her face very close to his and expressed some words of encouragement.

I asked Dr. Jeffries, "How many patients are scheduled for today?" because it was such a late start.

"I do not want to check the schedule because it would only make me frustrated. I want a clear head and get in my Zen mode when I walk in the exam room with the patient." Dr. Jeffries said, "I'm going to take control of the power in this interview. Unfortunately, this is going to be like Jurassic Park. There are raptors on the island; at night all the other dinosaurs get docile, but the raptors probe defenses for weakness. Watch for when the patient wrestles control of the interview from me." All of this occurred before we even walked in the room.

When we walked in the room, the patient was in a wheelchair facing from the curtains towards the two chairs on the opposite wall. The patient instructed Dr. Jeffries, "Empty my belongings off one of the chairs."

"No, I'll sit right next to it." Dr. Jeffries started by saying, "I'm going to give you a copy of your urodynamic study because I know you keep notebooks with all kinds of data." Dr. Jeffries then turned to the keyboard, sitting there until the end of the interview.

The patient was silent for a short time but then interrupted him to say, "It does leak," despite the fact that Dr. Jeffries reported there was no leakage on urodynamic studies. The patient went on to say, "It leaks when I cough or move. It happens four to six times a day."

Dr. Jeffries said, "Your bladder has shrunk to 250 mL."

"When I had those urodynamic studies, I started hollering and screaming because the pain intensity was so severe. The other doctor reported the comfortable volume limit of my bladder when he did previous urodynamic studies." The patient talked about the pain for a while.

Dr. Jeffries became quiet, and she was doing all the talking, "My bladder looks like an alien. I've seen pictures of my bladder." Dr. Jeffries continued sitting in the chair with his legs crossed. He listened for about twenty minutes and then interjected, "And that brings us to what can be done."

The patient replied, "I reflect, pray, reflect, pray."

Dr. Jeffries went on to explain, "High pressure in the bladder can damage the kidneys, and high pressure-causing reflux can also damage the kidneys. You told me you were worried about dialysis."

The patient changed the subject back to meds. "Previous doctors told me, 'This will work.' Nothing ever worked," and at that point she had her hands folded as Jesus is typically portrayed in the garden of Gethsemane. When I glanced over, I noticed that Dr. Jeffries had his hands in identical, mirroring position held closely together in front of his mouth. Following that, Dr. Jeffries put his fist on his chin in the thinker position and all this time the patient was producing a large amount of words describing mostly bladder spasms. At one point, the patient took her fist and smashed it into the other hand creating a forceful impact, trying to describe the pain associated with the spasm.

Dr. Jeffries was trying to work with her but she interrupted, saying, "I have constipation and diverticulitis, and I had impacted bowel. The pain is so bad. I do a lot of research." She repeated this phrase about doing a lot of research about ten times in the course of the interview. She followed that statement with, "What I'm thinking is, I'm not a doctor. I am a *me*. I don't think surgery would be helpful."

Dr. Jeffries tried to describe the ileovesicostomy[1] and said, "Of course it could never be a guarantee."

She interrupted and said, "I've got leak."

He said, "The goal is to increase the bladder capacity and decrease the pressure in the bladder and that will help to decrease the leakage. There's a trade-off between medications," and then gave a verbal physiologic explanation.

The patient responded by saying, "My experience is I know what I'm doing." She went on to explain, "Because of the scoliosis I take a lot of fiber and oats. I'm a lab experiment in trying to avoid medication."

Dr. Jeffries tried to acknowledge her concerns, "I appreciate the fact that the scoliosis causes some of the constipation."

She immediately came back, "There are many learned men, but I know my body and I know the research. I'm not a surgical candidate."

Dr. Jeffries said, "Surgery would be challenging, but the thing that scares me the most is the heart problems and lung problems. Those would be risky options. I could just revise your stoma."

The patient jumped on him verbally saying, "I just had that done." He tried to explain what it was, and she said, "I just had it done at University of Elsewhere."

He said, "Usually they don't use a catheter through that type of stoma."

"I do it anyway. My first problem started after becoming sexually active at 17 years old. I have three different sources of back pain. The onset of the issues began after my children were born. Then the onset of my issues was after I had the sling. I do research and talk to people who are a lot smarter than me, but I'm way up there." She then embarked on a monologue about, "what I'm thinking" and then she threw out there, "No one's talking to me . . . what is my renal function?"

Dr. Jeffries said, "I don't have any lab data. You refused to get worked up last time."

She replied, "I want to know how close I am to dialysis."

"You would need to see a nephrologist."

"I've already seen two of them, and I'm not a candidate for dialysis because my veins aren't good enough."

Dr. Jeffries recommended a medication for now, "because it would take the bladder neck and relax the body of the bladder, decrease the pressures, but it does run the risk of constipation."

The patient replied, "I do thorough research. Write the name of the medicine and give it to me and I'll look it up. The last time they tried to use medication I had a racing heartbeat to the point where I felt like I might stroke out. I've got some anxiety that I'm not a candidate for dialysis." The patient then said, "I haven't shared this with you, but I'm an ordained minister. I don't get blown out of shape by bad news. I want to know how close to dialysis I am," going into an extensive discussion, talking about the television show *House*,[2] and how she was watching the television show. "No one has given me a diagnosis and so I kept checking the symptoms off and, even though it's a fictitious show," implying she was making her own diagnosis, "my urine is light brown."

Dr. Jeffries said, "You lost a kidney."

"Where did it go?" and "I don't have much of an appetite – I lost weight."

"You're starving and didn't know it."

"I lost 41 pounds."

Dr. Jeffries was sitting with his arms crossed and his legs doubly crossed, not saying much. "When did you last see a nephrologist?"

"What's the difference between a nephrologist and a urologist?" When he explained that to her, she said, "You told me something I didn't know." The conversation proceeded and the patient said, "The nephrologist told me to get rid of the bacteria."

"That's not possible with a catheter in place. There is an important difference between infections and colonization, and he would prefer to be free of infection."

"I'm not to take any more antibiotics. When you take antibiotics you're selecting for resistant bacteria. I know. My previous urologist told me, since I'm not a candidate for dialysis, I need to flush my kidneys, so I drink a lot of water. My kidney is only about 40 percent functioning. Nobody listens to me anyway."

Dr. Jeffries told her she can put the papers in her file, and she verbally confronted him saying, "Don't generalize me."

Then Dr. Jeffries said, "The nephrologist was passionate, but he also wants to be realistic. It is like trying to get bacteria out of the garbage can," and then tried to backpedal the garbage can metaphor. Dr. Jeffries was paged and so he tried to wind up the interview. He was standing up, pushing the pager button every time the pager went beep. They had another extended discussion regarding antibiotics where the patient essentially wouldn't let him leave the room. He suggested an infectious disease specialist.

"We had those people." She talked about not having a functioning kidney, kept using the word, "no," then "No" in a louder tone of voice, and then said to Dr. Jeffries, "You guys are eggheads. My research shows that is all I need to do is concern myself with – I don't want any more medications. I don't want to discuss antibiotics. I don't want to discuss surgery. I know my body is ravaged by surgery. The reason I am here is to find out the level of kidney failure I have."

"Urodynamic studies aren't able to tell that."

She replied, "Well that's what I signed the papers for."

Dr. Jeffries said out loud, "No, no, no."

The patient echoed back, "No, no, no."

"Do you need help getting out of the room?"

I glanced at the clock. Dr. Jeffries spent an hour in the room with this patient. Carmen had to go back in the room and she got stuck in there another 15 minutes. Dr. Jeffries wanted to see his next patient, but he said to me, "I don't go by that route again." He essentially ran past the open door trying to get to his computer to find information to see the next patient.

Arthur Frank, in the *Wounded Storyteller*, insists that the body narrates itself and describes medical practice as "biomedical colonization." Although there is a pejorative tone to his nomenclature, this last vignette demonstrates how the illness narrative derails the healing ritual by not allowing the doctor to create the diagnosis narrative. To use Frank's own nomenclature, this patient is caught in a "chaos narrative," unable to be healed because she is preventing performance of the healing ritual. Dr. Jeffries anticipated this clinical encounter would be "painful." For me, it was painful to watch. There was none of the typical intimacy, trust, sharing, and shared goals I was used to seeing as part of daily life in the clinic.

The second case study I use to illustrate when the healing ritual fails is written by Susan Greenhalgh, *Under the Medical Gaze: Facts and Fictions of Chronic Pain* (Greenhalgh 2001). Very similar to the clinical vignette described earlier, the author-patient in her auto-ethnography begins by describing the tasks of the clinician within clinical encounters in a section called "How Medicine Works":

> The clinician's first task is to turn the person who comes into his office into an object of medical scrutiny: a patient.
>
> Second, the clinician must translate the disorganized details of the patient's suffering body into the "scientific facts" of the case – the diagnosis, prognosis, and treatment plan – and weave them together into a compelling story about what is wrong and what must be done to right it.
>
> Third, the doctor must convince the patient that the story is true, objective, and efficacious. That is, he must persuade the patient that the story is complete and error-free, unaffected by his values and interests, and will work to ease her pain.
>
> Fourth and finally, he must put the prescribed treatment into effect to improve on the suffering body by alleviating the symptoms of the illness he has diagnosed (which may or may not be what ails the patient).
>
> These four phases might be called those of patient construction, storytelling, persuasion, and treatment.
>
> (Greenhalgh 2001: 26–27)

This contemporary summary of the healing ritual is identical to the ritual portrayed in my ethnographic data. The one error is when she states, "*the illness* he has *diagnosed* [emphasis added]." Of course, the distinction of diagnosing a disease and diagnosing an illness is the major theme of this book. This goes all the way back to W.H.R. Rivers who realized *diseases* are *diagnosed*. Greenhalgh goes on to illustrate a firsthand account of how this ritual fails. Although she interprets her data in a different way, I will use her data to support the argument in my research.

After multiple attempts at finding "Doctor Right" and failing, "S" met "Dr. K," who was empathetic and caring as well as attending to the diagnostic investigation. The diagnosis proclaimed was "psoriatic arthritis." Eventually, "S" rejects this diagnosis, setting up the case identical to the first vignette in this chapter. Following that, "S" moves to the West Coast and consults a renowned doctor, Dr. D, who does an elaborate clinical encounter and proclaims five diagnoses: psoriatic arthritis, osteoarthritis, degenerative joint disease, fibromyalgia, and scoliosis. What ensues is a dramatic farce masquerading for medical care. "S" insists on tracking her own symptoms and reporting them as "data," which Dr. D discounts, upsetting "S" because she believes Dr. D doesn't respect her intellect (PhD in anthropology, a "doctor"). Instead, he collects his own "data" and begins prescribing medications with toxic side effects based on the diagnosis of fibromyalgia. The relationship is bumpy and the drama escalates, eventually ending with fury directed to the doctor for all the damage he did. This case illustrates the second major cause of failure of the healing ritual: misdiagnosis. Using my positionality as a doctor, Dr. D is a quack – unprofessional and dangerous because of his blind faith in his own ability to diagnose fibromyalgia. After tremendous suffering, "S" returns to Dr. K who treats her for psoriatic arthritis. "S" also enters psychotherapy and avails herself of a Kleinmanesque "re-storying" of past events (Greenhalgh 2001).

This case illustrates two healing rituals. The first failed because S. was not persuaded the diagnosis of psoriatic arthritis was correct. The second failed because the diagnosis of fibromyalgia was bogus. This extant ethnographic record explains what can be done if the patient does not accept the diagnostic narrative – find a different doctor. We typically call this a second opinion.

When the healing ritual fails, patients are vocal about telling their illness narratives. In fact, I think that the vast majority of the time, the healing ritual works, but this is the "unmarked" category of what is recorded by medical anthropologists. The failures are the "marked" category and are simply easier to find and record. I believe this sampling error is the major reason my findings are different from other anthropologists in the "narrative" healing literature.

Another example when the healing ritual did not meet the needs of the patient

Even when there is no cure, patients seem to need to be in a relationship with a doctor. This next example demonstrates how Dr. Stein embarked on a healing relationship with a new patient. Although Dr. Stein offered no cure, the patient was instructed to follow up. Because this was the first time Dr. Stein met the patient, the clinical encounter was devoid of Dr. Stein's dry wit, yet at the end of the visit the patient thanks the doctor.

Dr. Stein signaled to begin the next presentation, "Okay."
Dr. Williamson said, "This is a tough one." They reviewed all of the documents together. Dr. Williamson said, "He had a robotic cystoprostatectomy. The patient was initially scheduled for a prostate sparing surgery, but on frozen section in the operating room there was a positive margin

of bladder cancer in the prostate. The patient is upset; now he has incontinence and is wearing a condom catheter at night and has erectile dysfunction." It was extremely complex history. They reviewed the paper chart from Benedict Hospital as well as University of Elsewhere.

Dr. Stein said, "I don't understand why he came here."

"He left Benedict Hospital and Dr. Kilpatrick and went to University of Elsewhere where they offered him a sling, but he had two episodes of sepsis and has been followed up by urologists. He was treated with two weeks of ceftriaxone. He's just not happy with everything."

"He had outcome expectations," said Dr. Jeffries.

"He keeps asking why."

"He had irrational expectations."

Dr. Stein said, "He needs to go to a place where they know how to do robotic surgery – not Benedict Hospital."

Dr. Williamson said, "The final pathology didn't show any cancer in the prostate, but they did have the frozen section."

When we went in the room, the patient was obviously quite tense. Dr. Stein concentrated fully on the patient, making good eye contact, and he asked very specific questions about how much incontinence he is having and how much erectile dysfunction he's having. Dr. Stein then said, "Urology is a small specialty. Everybody knows everyone else. I've worked with all your previous doctors. I know the doctors at Benedict Hospital and I know the doctors at University of Elsewhere."

The patient said, "I just want to get on with life as usual. It is so frustrating." The frustration he mentioned was having to wear a diaper, having to do the self-catheterization. There was a long discussion about using a 16 French catheter versus a 14 French catheter, trying to flush out the mucus. One doctor told him he didn't have to do it; the other doctor and Dr. Stein said that he needs to flush out the mucus so he doesn't get a mucous plug that causes the incontinence at night. "I'm tired of wetting the bed and having to clean sheets, and during the day sometimes I wear two pairs of underwear." They had an extensive discussion regarding erectile dysfunction. "I've tried everything – Viagra, Cialis, vacuum pump, different formulations of penile injections – one injection caused pain. Right now, I'm getting a special pharmacy to the mix my injections. It's frustrating for me to hear that I have to cath myself every four hours. I'm only 51 years old, and it's frustrating."

Dr. Stein asked, "Do you want a penile implant? The penile implant might actually help with the incontinence because it causes a little bit of compression on the urethra."

The patient said, "That's what my original doctor told me, but one of the subsequent urologists told me it wasn't true."

"So two of three doctors told you that?" Dr. Stein offered suppressive antibiotics multiple times during the interview but each time said, "I don't recommend it, but it is available. I would lean against it." There was an implied non-recommendation for it. Dr. Stein summarized what was different but possible that he could do. "You need to see the doctor from the University or me, but [you] don't need both."

The patient said, "I live and work on the east side of town. I'll schedule follow-up with you." This was relatively long discussion. Both Dr. Stein and the patient were highly educated about dealing with these complications – the patient from his vast experience and Dr. Stein from working with these patients. They covered a lot of ground quickly.

There was also a discussion of the neo-bladder, how the attached ureter failed and he had to have repeat surgery. The patient asked, "What about an artificial sphincter?"

"That's more invasive than the sling." The problem with the sling was that he would certainly have to cath himself.

One of the more interesting things was after the office visit both Dr. Stein and the patient were standing at the appointment counter and the patient said, "Thanks. It helped."

It was such an intense feeling being in the room, I actually skipped the next patient. Dr. Stein saw the next patient without me. I asked Dr. Williamson, who did not go in with next patient either, what he thought about the patient. He said, "The patient was depressed. It was hard that he went from doctor to doctor and now is with us. We just have to take care of it. The most important part is to be honest. You don't want to lead him down that path," referring to the path of hope that it might get better, because it might not get better.

Notice the lack of the typical healing ritual structure – either for acute care or for the chronic care of the type that Dr. Spangler provides. I will return to these two cases during my concluding remarks. I think both of these cases have important theoretical implications.

Notes

1   An ileovesicostomy is a surgical procedure where the surgeon uses the tissue at the end of the small intestine to create a pouch that urine can drain into safely.
2   *House M.D.* is a drama/mystery television series (2004–2012). The main character is a doctor who specializes in diagnostic medicine for solving puzzling cases.

References

Greenhalgh, S. 2001. *Under the Medical Gaze*. Berkeley: University of California Press.

Mattingly, Cheryl. 1998. *Healing Dramas and Clinical Plots: The Narrative Structure of Experience.*Cambridge: Cambridge University Press.

Part IV

The body politic

The body politic or the social narrative was not the major focus of the research; I cannot pretend to discuss the body politic comprehensively because of the vastness of the topic. But it would be reasonable to report aspects of the body politic that did emerge in the data to provide validity by "triangulation." The body politic is the context within which the observations of the cultural body were gathered. Context is important for understanding. Context shapes the cultural practices of the office visits and treatments I was hoping to portray. Only the portions of the body politic that were readily apparent in my data are included here. I will discuss two major categories: (1) the business of medicine and (2) overdiagnosis and overtreatment, before concluding with a couple comments relating this research to the issues discussed.

These are contrasting perspectives. Consider how I described healing relationships and now I am going to discuss business relationships. The two coexist. Also, the emphasis on diagnosis could not be more apparent, but now I am going to discuss "overdiagnosis." Again, there is a dialectical tension that connects coexisting perspectives.

14 The business of medicine

Most people will accept that there is a business side to the practice of medicine. It is a contractual, exchange enterprise and it is easy to observe the business aspects of any medical setting (Davidoff 1998; Fins 2007; Pellegrino 1999). Medicine as a business also was apparent in my data. Kenneth Starr framed this question in his sweeping history of medicine in America, concluding with a poignant question: "Another key issue will be the boundary between medical and business decisions; when both medical and economic considerations are relevant, which will prevail and who will decide?" (Starr 1982: 447).

Advertising

Advertising is sometimes at the level of the individual physician, but in the geographic area of the field site, it is very frequently advertising at the health system level through print ads, radio and television ads, billboard ads, and endorsements. Five major health systems have well formulated branding campaigns that are easily recognized by color, slogan, and logo. If you stand in front of the downtown office of a cancer institute, there are two banners attached to every single streetlight, hanging vertically in a 1' x 4' rectangular blue fabric. On one side, the banner read "Hear Cancer," and on the other side it read "Think Cancer Institute." The total effect was a visual avenue leading you from one site to the other straight through the heart of the medical campus. The colors coordinated with the badges the physicians wore on their white coats, the artwork, the surface materials on the buildings, and so forth. The advertising worked so well that the urology practice struggled to obtain patients with other urological diagnoses. Internists want to refer to a urologist for general problems but won't refer patients to the urology department at Connaught because they associate it with cancer. One of the senior staff quoted the internist as saying, "Where do we send [kidney] stones?" The referral patterns were so deeply affected that an internist associated Dr. Jeffries's practice only with cancer, not realizing he also had a general urologic practice.

On another occasion, one of the administrators at Connaught called about a mailed advertisement for screening. "If someone wants to respond to the advertising, but had no insurance, they would be referred to financial services and then we could see them after that." This community outreach to increase market share is highly controversial, as I will discuss later.

As discussed in Chapter 11, every resident craves surgical experience as a marker of competence. Because of their educational debts, they attempt to make themselves marketable by learning the latest technology. Consider how revealing the following comment by one of the residents actually is: "Every surgeon wants training with robotics because patients perceive that the newest technology is the best and assume a surgeon trained with that technology is better. Actually, the reverse is true . . . unless you surpass the learning curve and develop expertise, the less technology is probably safer."

The following email, one of a biweekly series I received throughout the last part of my fieldwork, corroborates this resident's comment:

FW: Da Vinci Robotic Program Update 11-30
From: L Sayer
Date: November 30, 2012 4:34:53 PM
Subject: Da Vinci Robotic Program Update 11-30
Good afternoon,

Great News! We are in the news! We have been working with the Maplewood media department to get the word out about the new single site cholecystectomy and the [local newspaper] published the press release in yesterdays [sic] edition! Thanks to Mr. Wilder for his support in expediting the article. It is very exciting to see Maplewood Community Hospital in print. Kudos to Drs. Matthews and Marshall for already completing 3 of these surgeries and Dr. Howell who is very close to that goal. We are still waiting to hear from the Free Press and we are also looking at re-writing the article with a slightly more business angle for possible publication in Krain's.

To read the article, hold down the control button and click the following link:

Maplewood Da Vinci used in single incision surgery

www.hometownlife.com/article/202210596/BUSINESS/21158745/Mapelwood-s-da-Vinci-used-single-incision-surgery?odyssey=mod|newswell|text| s

On another publicity note, I was approached by Phyllis Grover from Public Relations this week regarding doing a segment on the single site surgery. Drs. Matthews and Marshall have agreed to speak and we are contacting their patients to possible speak as well

regarding their surgical experience. I guess good news
does travel fast.

We continue to grow and increase our numbers. We will
wrap up November with 85 total cases. Our original goal
for 2012 was 90, which we will surpass easily. We have
gotten in a few new supplies including the long has-
san trocar that so many of you have requested to use as
the camera port, and the D-Help scope defogger/cleaner/
heater system. Both are working great. We are waiting
to hear from the gas sterilizer company for a date for
the install of the new Ster-ad. This will help tremendously with scope sterilization turnover.

Please continue to call, text or see me with any questions or concerns regarding the Robotic program. I'm
here to help.

Thank You for supporting our Robotic Program!
Darlene Grady RN, BSN
Robotic Coordinator
Maplewood Community Hospital
Maplewood Mobile 704-555-2974
Cell 704-555-3397

This email is an example of "indication creep." Medical technology corpo-
rations designed the Da Vinci surgical system for a specific surgical problem
and it works well. To offset the expense, it is used for other procedures
(it creeps into general use), replacing technology that is a fraction of the
Da Vinci expense . . . without any evidence that there is any benefit to the
patient. The healthcare industrial complex contributes to the "healthcare
crisis" by encouraging overtreatment. Referring to the Da Vinci robotic
surgery system, Shannon Brownlee calls this the "medical-technology arms
race" (Brownlee 2007: 163).

A general surgery resident confirmed that the hospital does put subtle
pressure on doctors to use the Da Vinci robotic surgical system once it is
purchased. He said that for most general surgery procedures it is suboptimal
because you can't get the sense of touch you would with a laparoscopic or
open procedure. He said, "The system was originally designed for surgery
in confined spaces, such as the pelvis, but now I'm being trained to use it
for general surgery procedures in the abdomen, such as a cholecystectomy"[1]
(Beck 2013).

Patient satisfaction

Business and healthcare systems compete. One measure of competition is
on "quality scores." Hospital Care Quality Information from the Consumer Perspective (HCAHPS) is a national, standardized, 27-item, publicly

reported survey recognized by the Center for Medicare and Medicaid Services (CMS), and multiple other divisions of the Department of Health and Human Services. The Patient Protection and Affordable Care Act of 2010 (P.L. 111–148) specifically included HCAHPS performance in the calculation of the value-based incentive payment in the Hospital Value-Based Purchasing program, beginning with discharges in October 2012. During my fieldwork at the clinic, the screensaver (on 18 computers) cycled through the specific questions on the survey related to nurses and doctors. It was like subliminal advertising for the employees so that the health system could be more competitive on the quality score.

The Hospital Consumer Assessment of Healthcare Providers and Systems (HCAHPS score) determines "value-based incentives" and includes the following two questions:

1   How often did doctors listen carefully to you?
2   How often did doctors explain things to you in a way you could understand?

These questions are "patient satisfaction" scores. Typically, doctors revile these scores because they conflate "quality" with "satisfaction," which sometimes conflict (Jones-Nosacek 2015; Mehta 2015). Another federal government program that uses patient satisfaction scores to enhance reimbursement is the Patient Centered Medical Home (PCMH). Evidence that this program improves quality of care is controversial, but it has entered into the lexicon of medical practice.

Dr. Stein started joking around a little bit, specifically in regard to patient-centered outcomes research. Dr. Stein said, referring to the patients, "I just tell them they are supposed to listen to me."
The administrator commented, "That's not a very patient-centered approach."
Dr. Stein continued, saying, "What do you mean my patients don't understand? I don't care if they understand as long as they do as I say." At this point, he was joking about the patient-centered outcomes research, but the joke wasn't funny, because his statement was consistent with times when I saw the doctor making the diagnosis and deciding what is appropriate treatment prior to entering the exam room.

Although Dr. Stein was contradicting political correctness, I eventually realized that he was correct with regard to the interpretation of my results and the healing ritual. Doctors perform a risk assessment and review the anatomical and pathophysiological dimensions of the problem before going in the exam room to see the patient. The healing ritual occurs only if this cognition is shared and accepted by patient and doctor. Far from making the patient into an object or diseased organ, this is the process for all enculturation. Although politically incorrect, the cultural practice benefits the patient. The following illustration speaks more directly to the ultimate goal of benefiting the patients.

> There was a quiet moment and Dr. Stein sat down, eating lunch. He was talking to me and I shared with him my prior work related to hierarchy in medical education. He seemed very interested in that and then said, "There are people higher than me." I commented that as chair of his department there weren't too many. He responded to my comment, "The patients are the boss."
>
> Later that same day, Dr. Jeffries said aloud, "He is the most important person," and nodded in the direction of the patient he just saw.
>
> Marsha looked at me and said, "There, you've heard it out of both of the horses' mouths."

Both Dr. Stein and Dr. Jeffries verbalized that the patient is their "boss." The drive to provide better care, the best care possible, occurs in the context of doctors who truly care about their patients. It does not mean that they have to abandon the basic tenets of medical practice. It does mean that they re-evaluate experiences of the difficult partial nephrectomy of the patient who was taking aspirin. It does mean figuring out how to offer active surveillance for prostate cancer when there is no easy way to do it. Consider the following interaction:

> As Dr. Jeffries was leaving the clinic, I asked him about a comment he made earlier in the afternoon, to no one in particular, while approaching the exam room, "This will be like pounding my head against the wall." I asked him what he meant by that. He said, "The patient comes in every six months with an elevated PSA in the range of 10 to 16. He is a very high-risk patient, being African American and elderly. Every six months we go over the rationale for doing a biopsy. I believe it is my due diligence to recommend a prostate biopsy to this patient. I do that every six months only to have the patient tell me, 'I don't want to know.' Despite my offer to biopsy his prostate every single time I see him, he tells me the same thing, but in the end, I work for him."

The combination of "banging his head against a wall," a painful experience, striving for "due diligence," and recognizing he works for the patient, I suggest, is the equivalent of the clinician engaging in self-reflective interpretation of the interests, biases, and emotions that underlie his own model of patient care. This is a component of Arthur Kleinman's Patient Explanatory Model. I found confirmatory evidence for this in comments from the epidemiologist researcher-clinician who works with Dr. Jeffries:

> He thinks active surveillance is the right thing to do for certain patients. He is a surgeon and, yes, he loves to do surgery. But he also doesn't want to create harm where there isn't any need to, and he does a good job of

following people. Another thing that's come up in our discussions that's given as a reason for not recommending active surveillance is the concern that people won't follow up in time. Again, getting to the medical-legal aspects, you know if they don't [surgically remove the prostate], in every three, four, six months or whatever you decide is the time they need to follow up for their PSA or they won't have their next biopsy in 12, 18 months . . . Are you then liable? Because he didn't take it [the prostate gland] out right when you had the chance?

Dr. Jeffries said, "Yeah that is a concern."

Active surveillance has no standard of care, yet the standard of care is the legal definition of malpractice. Yet Dr. Jeffries wants to do the right thing.

I believe this demonstrates the underlying professionalism and the value of service to patients that is part of the medical culture. Drs. Stein and Jeffries enjoy great patient satisfaction scores because they meet the basic needs of patients – not because they listen carefully to patients. Based on the healing ritual I described, the patient satisfaction questions are incorrectly phrased. A better way to measure "quality" is to ask the patient the following closely related questions:

1   Was the doctor careful enough to make an accurate diagnosis?
2   Did the doctor persuade you that the diagnosis was correct?

A better measure of quality may be, "Did the doctor make the correct diagnosis?" This is certainly relevant to the data in this study. Avoidable diagnostic errors account for 160,000 deaths annually and approximately $10 billion in malpractice payouts (1986–2010; Landro 2013). Measuring quality in today's healthcare marketplace is very controversial. I believe that the core function of a doctor is to name the existential threat; every other aspect of healthcare flows from that "root cause" decision. I believe making the correct diagnosis and successfully performing the healing ritual should be a measure of "physician added value" – a better measure than patient satisfaction. During my fieldwork, patient satisfaction was mentioned rarely and in an offhand manner, it was never considered as part of "the work of the physician" – that distinction was reserved for the extraordinary efforts put into diagnosis.

Physician incentives

Although health systems compete for market share, doctors are reimbursed based on the amount of clinical activity and revenue they generate. Dr. Jeffries asked Dr. Stein what he thought about robotic surgery versus open surgery and Dr. Stein replied very quickly, "I want to send my kids to college."

Similarly, Dr. Jeffries was seeing a patient that had a history of back problems. It turned out that the patient had four neurosurgery procedures. Dr.

Jeffries was surprised, "You mean you had another neurosurgery since the last time I saw you?" There was a lot of surprise; he elevated his tone of voice and then Dr. Jeffries said, "What's going on . . . is this neurosurgeon putting his kids through college at your expense?"

In many ways, subtle incentives create a framework for clinical practice. At times, they are mutually re-enforcing. Consider the following except from an interview with a clinician extremely familiar with my field site. She begins talking about developing a program related to active surveillance for prostate cancer.

"But when you ask Dr. Jeffries to think about urologists in the community and what would be some of the barriers to doing this, of course, medical legal is a big one. Let's say the person does develop aggressive cancer and goes back and sues you. Urologists don't want to be in that situation. Right now there's no . . . let's say negative consequences for the urologist. In fact there may be positive downstream consequences for the urologist to do the surgery. You know then you've gotta repair the incontinence and impotence. So they're a patient for life. So there's a monetary and financial rewards for the individual patient care as well as negating the fear of the lawsuits. Because you've done what standard of care is whereas active surveillance is not standard of care yet, or may never be. And then we got into, what we found in our study was that the whole robotic thing is 'phwew.' "

Although both Dr. Jeffries and Dr. Stein joked about making money by doing more surgery, I never felt they influenced patients to "rush into surgery." In fact, the exact opposite occurred. I witnessed a lengthy discussion about active surveillance (delaying surgery) and the time invested in providing appropriate informed consent, only to fall victim to our cultural model of "cancer – cut it out."

Billing and insurance

Businesses have to measure productivity and monitor cash flow. In medical systems, this is done with "documentation and billing." Again, if you see Medicare or Medicaid patients, CMS standardizes the entire process by regulation, enforced by audit. Criminal penalties for fraud accrue to the individual physician. Clinical activity measured by billing determines physician compensation. When Dr. Jeffries was working with Dr. Williamson, he said, "There are templates [in the electronic medical record] for that."

"I can't believe this. I just had a complex discussion with the patient about elevated PSA. I took extra effort to do shared decision-making. There's no template in this electronic medical record for an increased PSA."

Marsha replied, "Why don't you ask the electronic medical record team to generate one for you. Their job is to make your job easier."

Dr. Jeffries said, "Yeah, the electronic medical record team is all about helping out the doctors," very sarcastically.

"Dr. Jeffries, I think you should try yoga. That's what I recommend."

The cause of Dr. Jeffries frustration was that in his mind, he had done a lot of work explaining a complex medical choice to a patient, but the template in the electronic health record didn't reflect that amount of work which meant that he wouldn't get paid for his effort.

Similarly, Dr. Jeffries referred to the software architecture while working at the documentation countertop:

Dr. Jeffries was working with Dr. Williamson, saying, "There are templates for this diagnosis that are comprehensive and fulfill all the criteria for Level 4 billing."[2]

Dr. Jeffries was distracted by a phone call, and Dr. Williamson was using the electronic medical record, choosing different radio buttons to click pre-defined choices in the database that would eventually be assembled into a clinical progress note. He said to me, "I object to progress notes written with electronic health records because it's too much. I like to type with free text."

While Dr. Williamson was working, Dr. Jeffries was on the phone but leaned over and said to Dr. Williamson, "If you're going to document, you do it my way." Dr. Jeffries then showed Dr. Williamson how to use the software template by walking him through how to use the template in the software. "It's not kidney pain, dude." Dr. Jeffries demonstrated how to navigate through the medical record using only mouse clicks – click, click, click – the two of them standing side by side as they completed the progress note together.

This is an example where the input to the electronic health record is important, not for patient care, but for billing purposes. It is widely recognized by doctors that the electronic health record is useful for storing data and generating billing documentation, but not helpful for actually taking care of patients.[3] I mentioned earlier that the database architecture records isolated facts without a narrative structure. Simply recording a series of "elements" justifies billing. For instance, there is no "click" for an emotion, chronology, or cause and effect – all critical elements of narrative.

Dr. Stein did something very similar during an office visit. Dr. Stein turned his attention to the computer screen and essentially spoke out loud each word that he typed in to the medical record talking throughout the entire documentation process. At one point, Dr. Stein confirmed with a medical student a fact that was part of the documentation. He then showed the medical student a very detailed checkbox history and physical and told the medical student he could click the radio button that said detailed/reviewed turning to the medical student, saying, "These papers will be scanned into the medical record and that will prove that I reviewed them." He got to the part about documenting the physical exam he was still talking out loud and stated, "prostate enlarged, grade 2, 60 grams without nodules." He then moved on to the assessment and while typing said, "Ninety-year-old male, digital rectal exam non-suspicious, do not recommend biopsy." He then turned to the medical student and said, "Now the computer will just generate a chart note," and Dr. Stein made a sound like "zoom zoom" as the database elements in the electronic health record were compiling the note. After showing the note to the medical student, he said, "Now we want to generate a consult thank you." He pushed a button, which generated a templated letter in the computer. He deleted the salutation of "dear colleague" and entered in the primary care physician's full name, checking on the spelling.

Even more important for urologists is to bill for procedures and surgeries – these have a high reimbursement rate. This requires identifying the proper ICD-9 code. I observed Barb and Dr. Patel having a long conversation, going over codes about the surgery he was going to do. He tried to explain, "It is for a different reason. We can't bill for total revision – I'm going to do a revision and that has a different code. I'm only going to fix the reservoir [of an implantable erectile dysfunction device]. I don't know if there's a separate code for it, but the tubing comes from the reservoir . . . these codes irritate me." Barb asked a question and he answered saying, "Yes. The patient is very skinny. Originally, I put the tubes under the skin, but there is no fat. I may have to put under the muscle." He started pointing to his own body. In the end, Dr. Patel said, "Use the revision code."

While standing at the desk, Dr. Stein had a conversation with Charlene, the billing person, who had walked in and out of the clinic approximately five times during this particular session, more than any other time I've been in the clinic. Dr. Stein said to her, "I don't want you to think I'm going behind your back," and shared with her an email that he had initiated to someone else with billing expertise. He said, "You did say 585.76," and then named two more codes. "I did a 583.99 which correlates with unlisted bladder procedure or we could use 385.72 for an extended surgery. There is no code for laparoscopic cystectomy. I'll take the email and forward it to the billing person at the Maplewood site." While he was still in the hallway Charlene brought back a coding book with descriptions and Dr. Stein said, "There is no CPT code for a surgery that is done half laparoscopically and half open."

Big Pharma

Dr. Spangler takes into consideration whether the patient's insurance covers the specific chemotherapy agent before she even considers offering it to the patient. In this way, pharmaceutical companies and insurance companies are implicitly making medical decisions. Medicare is not allowed to negotiate pharmaceutical prices by law (Kantarjian et al. 2013). Our society seems to tolerate outrageous behavior by "Big Pharma" (Brody 2011; Gotzsche 2012; Outterson 2012; Ross 2008; Smith 2005; Spielmans 2010).

Corporate mergers

During my fieldwork, of the five major health systems in the geographic area, a for-profit corporation purchased one of the non-profit health systems and two non-profit health systems announced plans to merge. Healthcare in the United States is not becoming less expensive. The free-enterprise system and the "right" to healthcare are values that cannot be reconciled. The system is unsustainable in its current formulation. Doctors are highly aware of the multiple institutions and their relative market positions and politics.

Once, in the middle of a clinic session, Dr. Spangler went over to talk to Dr. Bridges across the charting room. She was talking about Valkyrie, the for-profit corporation who took over University Hospital, and talking about rumors that they wanted to take over Connaught also. She asked Dr. Bridges, "Is it true?"
He said, I sent an email to Eric at the Cleveland Clinic. "He's a man in touch with Valkyrie. They [Valkyrie] bought up several hospitals around them."
A different oncologist joined them. He came over to the cubicle and said, "Over the weekend I visited Johns Hopkins and saw the new hospital. It cost $1 billion."
Dr. Spangler asked, "Where did they get the money?"
"The Sheikh – they were trying to figure out which one of his 12 names to use as the name of the hospital. I got to tour the hospital the day before it opened so I was able to walk through the ICU, through all different parts of the hospital without any impediment at all."

During my fieldwork, I found little evidence that business demands prevailed in caring for patients. Subsequently, however, I find that American medicine has reached the tipping point to the extent that Kenneth Starr's rhetorical question is now relevant to current practice. By manipulating benefits, insurance companies are practicing medicine, or at least preventing doctors from treating life-threatening clinical situations. This problem is explained in Appendix B, when Dr. Spangler describes choice of chemotherapy. I routinely audio-record my conversations with insurance companies while seeking pre-authorization when I believe the patient's life is in danger and the insurance company withholds lifesaving therapy (such as insulin for a Type I diabetic patient). That alternative narrative, however, is beyond the scope of this ethnography.

Notes

1 Cholecystectomy is the name of the surgery to remove a gall bladder.
2 Level 4 indicates a higher reimbursement amount for this visit – achievable only if you have all the components of the medical history included in the electronic medical record.
3 This was confirmed by a doctor in the Dartmouth Healthcare system that made the remark when she found out the name of the software this institution used for the medical record. Others in the system routinely only use the "Assessment and Plan" portion of the computer-generated note because it is the only part that is recorded reflecting the doctor's thinking. The toggle buttons mentioned by Dr. Jeffries contain no chronology and no emotional choices, destroying much of the narrative functions of a history and physical.

References

Beck, Melinda. 2013. Study Doubts Value of Robotic Surgery. *Wall Street Journal*, February 20, 2013.

Brody, Howard. 2011. The Inverse Benefit Law: How Drug Marketing Undermines Patient Safety and Public Health. *American Journal of Public Health* 101(3).

Brownlee, Shannon. 2007. *Overtreated: Why Too Much Medicine Is Making Us Sicker and Poorer*. New York: Bloomsbury USA.

Davidoff, F. 1998. Medicine and Commerce. 2: The Gift. *Annals of Internal Medicine* 128(7):572–575.

Fins, J.J. 2007. Commercialism in the Clinic: Finding Balance in Medical Professionalism. *Cambridge Quarterly of Healthcare Ethics* 16(4):425–432; Discussion 439–442.

Gotzsche, G.P.C. 2012. Big Pharma Often Commits Corporate Crime, and This Must Be Stopped. *British Medical Journal* 345(e8462).

Jones-Nosacek, Cynthia. 2015. Treating Patients as Customers – Whom Does It Help? *Wisconsin Medical Journal* 114(6).

Kantarjian, Hagop M., et al. 2013. Cancer Drugs in the United States: *Justum Pretium* – the Just Price. *Journal of Clinical Oncology* 31(28).

Landro, Laura. 2013. The Biggest Mistake Doctors Make. *Wall Street Journal*, November 18, 2013.

Mehta, Shivan J. 2015. Ethics Case: Patient Satisfaction Reporting and Its Implications for Patient Care. *AMA Journal of Ethics* 17(7):616–621.

Outterson, K. 2012. Punishing Health Care Fraud: Is the GSK Settlement Sufficient? *New England Journal of Medicine* 367(12).

Pellegrino, E.D. 1999. The Commodification of Medical and Health Care: The Moral Consequences of a Paradigm Shift From a Professional to a Market Ethic. *Journal of Medicine Philosophy* 24(3):243–266.

Ross, J.S. 2008. Guest Authorship and Ghostwriting in Publications Related to Ofecoxib: A Case Study of Industry Documents From Rofecoxib Litigation. *JAMA* 299(15).

Smith, R. 2005. Medical Journals Are an Extension of the Marketing Arm of Pharmaceutical Companies. *PLoS Medicine* 2(5):e138.

Spielmans, G.I. 2010. From Evidence Based Medicine to Marketing Based Medicine: Evidence From Internal Industry Documents. *Bioethical Inquiry* 7(13).

Starr, Paul. 1982. *The Social Transformation of American Medicine*. New York: Basic Books.

15 Overdiagnosis and overtreatment

For the individual patient and doctor, one cultural model is "find cancer and cut it out." That seems the compassionate thing to do; cancer is, after all, quite scary. Even scarier is the following quote attributed to Dr. Otis Webb Brawley, now the chief medical officer for the American Cancer Society:

> We at Emory have figured out that if we screen 1,000 men at the North Lake Mall this coming Saturday, we could bill Medicare and insurance companies for $4.9 million in health care costs [for biopsies, tests, prostatectomies, etc.]. But the real money comes later – from the medical care the wife will get in the next three years because Emory cares about her man, and from the money we get when he comes to Emory's emergency room when he gets chest pain because we screened him three years ago.
>
> ... We don't screen anymore at Emory, once I became head of Cancer Control. It bothered me, though, that my P.R. and money people could tell me how much money we would make off screening, but nobody could tell me if we could save one life. As a matter of fact, we could have estimated how many men we would render impotent ... but we didn't. It's a huge ethical issue.
>
> (Brawley and Goldberg 2011)

Screening for prostate cancer with PSA has a legacy that will not go away. The following comments are by the primary care doctor epidemiologist that works with Dr. Jeffries:

> Well in our study we sent out, we had 380 surveys on prostate cancer treatment decision-making. Over half of patients chose surgery and 80 percent of them did robotic surgery. They were convinced that there are fewer side effects with robotic. And if you read the marketing materials for robotics, it's pretty much marketed that way. It doesn't say we have less side effects this way, but it's the most innovative and technologically advanced in order to minimize your side effects from the surgery. But do you know how much one of those machines cost?

We looked it up. And we were talking to Dr. Jeffries about that, and he was like, "yeah it takes a good five years of everyday use to pay one of those machines off." And yes, there is pressure that comes down from the hospital when they put out that kind of money, they want to see their machine used so they'll do all the marketing for you but they still want to see it used. So when you're, imagine you're in the office with the patient who says, "I have this cancer get it out of me." It has to be awfully tempting to say, "Oh, we can do that for you." Rather than, "Well, and you know it's sort of a low risk cancer. One of the options and I would recommend this one would be let's watch it for a while. Not that we won't eventually do surgery or we may not have to. There is . . ."

Overtreatment is one part of the healthcare crisis. Another part is overdiagnosis (Carter et al. 2015). Doctors act in the setting of the body politic, and in many ways, the conflict of societal values gets played out in what I consider to be the poster child, the first and most controversial case of overdiagnosis: PSA screening. There are astute clinicians that have already given the clarion call that prostate cancer is the tip of the iceberg; pulmonary embolism is currently being debated in the medical literature as an example of overuse in emergency department settings (Brownlee 2007; Welch et al. 2011). Shannon Brownlee also gives the following description at Johns Hopkins:

> The cancer center, by contrast, lures a better-insured clientele, in part because the disease itself is most common among Medicare recipients. Chemotherapy represents a major source of profit for any cancer center, because the hospital buys the drugs wholesale and permitted by Medicare and the state of Maryland to mark up the price by about 16 percent. Radiation therapy is also profitable. "There's an incentive to say we're not going to do psychiatry because we lose money," said Langbaum. "So we really should refuse to admit psychiatry patients and admit more surgery patients. The problem with that is this is a teaching institution, and we can't pick up and choose what we will take care of. So we try and develop programs that do make money to [be able to] run the programs that don't make money."
>
> In other words, Hopkins does what all hospitals must do: It uses the profits it makes on some patients to cross-subsidize the care of others. A hospital's "refuges of profit," as departments that make money are sometimes called.
>
> (Brownlee 2007: 81–82)

Throughout my entire medical career, I have been warned of the "demographic imperative," referring to aging baby boomers who will consume ever-larger segments of society's healthcare resources as they accumulate

chronic diseases and die. Dr. Spangler referred to the demographic imperative when one of the medical assistants told her one of the patients was
requesting a handicap-parking sticker, which required a doctor's signature.
Dr. Spangler looked at me and said, "It's not gonna help because all the
handicap parking spots are going to be taken. He won't be able get a handicap spot because everybody's getting older."

As men age, the chance that they have prostate cancer cells in the prostate
increases so that by the time they are ninety years old, there is an 80–90 percent probability prostate cancer cells are present. The next section relates
data reflective of conflict within the body politic regarding who and how
scientific medical information is interpreted and deployed.

The wife said, "I was reading in the newspapers that prostate cancer is a
slow growing cancer."

Dr. Spangler then said, "Yes, That was a big deal up there on Capitol Hill.
There is a lot of controversy about unnecessary treatment, but you talk
to two different people and one person will say 'it saved my life' and the
other personal will say 'that's totally crazy.' Some doctors don't think
that we should be screening with PSA . . . there was all that mess about
mammograms but we got that fixed – women are better advocates. PSA
is here, we might as well use it."

The "mess that got fixed" about mammograms was the United States Pre-
ventative Services Task Force (USPSTF) recommendation that women discuss getting a mammogram with their doctor, published on November 6,
2009. It created shock and anger, and eventually the USPSTF reversed the
recommendation because of political pressure, typified by then Representative Wasserman's appearance on CNN. In a broader context, mammograms
are extremely controversial (Meza 2015; Miller et al. 2014).

The Healthcare Effectiveness Data and Information Set (HEDIS) is a measure of performance on important dimensions of care and service. HEDIS
was developed and is maintained by the National Committee for Quality
Assurance (NCQA). One of the measures is breast cancer screening rate; it is
represented as a measure of quality with the assumption that breast cancer
screening should be done. Again, financial incentives for healthcare systems
are directly tied to these national measures of quality. However, compare
the USPSTF recommendation, Dr. Spangler's comments, and the following
summary from the Cochrane Library – the single best source of evidence-
based care:

It may be reasonable to attend for breast cancer screening with mammography, but it may also be reasonable not to attend, as screening has
both benefits and harms.

If 2000 women are screened regularly for 10 years, one will benefit
from the screening, as she will avoid dying from breast cancer.

At the same time, 10 healthy women will, as a consequence, become cancer patients and will be treated unnecessarily. These women will have either a part of their breast or the whole breast removed, and they will often receive radiotherapy, and sometimes chemotherapy.

Furthermore, about 200 healthy women will experience a false alarm. The psychological strain until one knows whether or not it was cancer, and even afterwards, can be severe.

www.cochrane.dk/screening/index-en.htm

Updated version states, "Mammography screening does not work and leads to substantial overdiagnosis."[1]

In the middle of my fieldwork, the USPSTF recommended against screening for prostate cancer with digital rectal exam or PSA. Again, this caused controversy. At a national conference with experts from all parts of the country, the topic came up for discussion. Recognizing the controversy, Dr. Stein attempted to initiate a discussion, saying, "You University guys," and at that point, the audience participation was enormous with people standing up and raising their hands trying to talk. The discussion ended in pandemonium.

Dr. Jeffries spoke vehemently against USPSTF recommendations because "The recommendations were being driven by trying to avoid overtreatment. Their recommendations are like sticking your head in the sand. The task force is just upset that we're over treating prostate cancer."

Despite the recommendation, Dr. Jeffries did not change his clinical practice; while speaking with patients he said, "You're due for your prostate cancer check today; you've had the blood work but I need to do the rectal exam. Most urologists do a gentle rectal exam, thank goodness, but that's part of your cancer screening." He would also remind patients when they were due for screening in the future. He is consistent with specialty guidelines:

> The American Urological Association (AUA) believes that the prostate-specific antigen (PSA) test, when used appropriately, provides clinicians with valuable information to aid in the diagnosis and treatment of prostate cancer. Currently, there is not a comparable test or diagnostic available for this purpose. In May 2012, the U.S. Preventive Services Task Force (USPSTF) issued final recommendations discouraging the use of the PSA test. The AUA strongly believes that the USPSTF, in disparaging the PSA test before a newer diagnostic is more readily available, does a great disservice to American men and may cause more harm than good.[2]

Dr. Spangler summarized it best: "All research is focused on the most important question, which is, we don't know what is indolent tumor and what is aggressive tumor."

Naturally, these disparate opinions cause confusion.

While the participants were discussing the issue of prostate cancer at the national urology conference I mentioned, Dr. Fields leaned over to me and said, "This prostate cancer stuff is like a shit-show. They're all experts up there and they can't agree." On another occasion, Dr. Smith told me,

> That's what I hate about urology and prostate cancer. It is very confusing. I understand the risk of harm and the risk of benefit of doing surgery for prostate cancer . . . incontinence and erectile dysfunction, surgical complications. You do so many surgeries to prevent one death from prostate cancer, but dying from prostate cancer is such a miserable experience, the last two years are just a total misery. You have to do it to so many people to prevent one actual case of aggressive prostate cancer. Dr. Stein is now using active surveillance much more commonly than he had done in the past.

This societal conflict is played out in the cultural body. Consider the following office visit:

The patient said, "I came to you for surgery because you are highly recommended. I did some online investigating about prostate cancer and read a lot about it and the different types of treatment options that were available. I have a lot of cancer in my family and I think I want surgery . . . I want to get rid of it before it spreads."

Dr. Stein then reviewed the biopsy report that was done on September 1, 2011, and reported that the Gleason score was 6. Dr. Stein said, "Each biopsy is given two scores, each score can be 3, 4 or 5, and so the Gleason score can range from 3+3 which equals 6, all the way up to 5+5, which equals 10. It could also be 3+4, which would be a 7, etc. Your prostate was fairly large and they had only 10 cores on your biopsy." He then drew a picture of the size of the core and indicated the size of the prostate with his hand motions. He summarize by saying, "There are two problems that occur in men as they get older with their prostate. One is that the size enlarges and the other one is that it can develop cancer. Only one of the 10 cores showed cancer and that core showed it was a Gleason 6. There is no indication that the cancer had spread outside the prostate."

The patient said, "I'm not that concerned about sexual functioning but my biggest concern is incontinence."

Dr. Stein then went into a lengthy explanation of possible incontinence from robotic surgery. He said, "Let me define good. We call good when the patient does not have to use the pad but may have small drops and has to wear a small absorbent pad in the underwear. That's just catch a few drops of urine if you cough or sneeze. You're young and there was not an extensive tumor so we would recommend a nerve sparing surgery.

I feel safe doing that. I want to wait at least six weeks after the biopsy so the inflammation is down, to make the surgery technically easier."

"Because you are young and healthy I would recommend one of two things: Either definitive surgery, which would be curative, or active surveillance. Active surveillance would be reasonable because I think there is a very small amount of tumor and it isn't very aggressive. If you chose active surveillance, I would recommend a repeat prostate biopsy with perhaps up to as many as 20 or 30 cores because of the large size of your prostate, to get a better sample. A sampling error is missing some of the prostate cancer."

"The other option is robotic surgery, where I'm sitting in a booth using levers and pedals and I have an assistant at the table who inserts the instruments. The incisions would be small and we put the prostate and a few lymph nodes in a plastic bag take them out of one of the incisions, which would have to be a bit larger in order to get the plastic bag with the tissue out of your body."

Dr. Stein then brought up again active surveillance saying, "No treatment is perfect. The surgery has problems with sexual functioning just not being as good and potential incontinence. About 95 percent of patients do not have problems with incontinence as I described it earlier but 5 percent might, and that's the reason to choose active surveillance. If it does happen to you, there are things we can do about it."

At this point the wife interjected and said, "His mother was diagnosed with cancer in her thirties and died in her forties and his father died of cancer, three uncles died of cancer, and I have to live with him and he will be crabby."

Dr. Stein replied, "So it would be difficult for you to wait."

The patient said, "Yes." He asked his wife if she had any concerns. She kept telling him it was up to him and he replied, "The decision involves you too because of the sexual functioning."

She said, "I'm getting old and don't care."

The patient turned to Dr. Stein and said, "Let's do it. Let's go ahead and schedule the surgery. I just want it taken care of."

Although Dr. Stein offered active surveillance as an alternative management plan to "cancer – cut it out," the patient reverted to surgery as his preference. Most urologists wouldn't even offer active surveillance.

The following transcript is from an interview with the clinician/epidemiologist who made the previous comments. She reflects on clinical situations such as these.

And we had an ACS grant on prostate cancer treatment decision-making. The results of that are leading us to, as well as what's been happening just in general in the world of prostate cancer, led us to the conviction that the really interesting area to study is active surveillance or watchful waiting. There was just this huge NIH panel last year on the need to study the offer and acceptance and adherence to active surveillance. So the timing has been really good for us to study those. So we started talking. And we met with him three or four times, just again to get his idea of what a urologist out there thinking about active surveillance. How do they think about? What would be some of the motivators and barriers to doing it? And he's . . . so he's teaching in the residency program, so you have to be on top of what's the latest out there. And so as far as recognizing who might be a good candidate for active surveillance and teaching that to the residents and then how do we follow them and what's the best protocol . . . there is no set protocol out there. So what would be a good protocol? He pretty much individualizes it, which is nice too.

He thinks active surveillance is the right thing to do for certain patients. I mean, that's the impression I get. I've never really asked him, but I think he said that. You know why be— yes he is a surgeon and yes, he loves to do surgery. But he also doesn't want to create harm where there isn't any need to and he doesn't really, he does a good job of following people. And now another thing that's come up in our discussions with him that we've seen in the literature and, um, that's given as a reason for not recommending active surveillance is the concern that people won't follow up in time. Again, getting to the medical legal aspects you know if they don't, in every three, four, six months or whatever you decide is the time they need to follow up for their PSA or they won't have their next biopsy in 12, 18 months. Are you then liable? Because he didn't take it out right when you had the chance. He said, you know, "yeah that is a concern." They fortunately have a good follow-up system and he, you really do have to screen the patients well to make sure that they understand how important it is to follow-up and that they are able to follow up. You know, transportation difficulties, insurance, all that. Although in this population Medicare is usually there, so that doesn't have as much of an effect on it.

And again, I only have two patients that are in this program with him and they, they are so happy that they are and that he, he does wait it out. I mean, I have one guy who, his PSA was going up just a little you know and he was getting a little nervous. I mean Dr. Jeffries said, "We'll just check it. Then instead of six months we're going to do three months. We'll keep an eye on it." And he's probably, he's only like 53 or 54. Any other urologist would just say, "I'm not risking it. I'm not risking it." But he's a smart guy and he did his homework too and said, "I'm not ready to deal with complications, so let's do it this way."

You know there is a lot of medical literature on watchful waiting but watchful waiting really was a different thing than active surveillance. Well, watchful waiting – active surveillance. Let me try it actually – active surveillance is low risk, low rise, Gleason score less than six, PSA less than 10, and stage less than 2A. so it took defined criteria. Watchful waiting never had that. Watchful waiting, tended to be more for in my opinion older folk whose life span was going to be limited anyway and so we'll just watch it while you're dying of other things. Active is more active, watchful waiting was definitely a passive sort of approach. It has its criteria I that should have protocols and it should be more standardized, although according to Dr. Jeffries, would be really hard to standardize it because it has to be individualized somewhat. I mean if you, I think that individualization still comes down to algorithms. You know yeah if you see the doubling time, if that's what you're choosing to watch, going up then you go for biopsy even though you weren't due for a biopsy for another six, 12 months. So yeah I mean it can all be algorithm'ed out. I'm not the best person to do that but I think Dr. Stein is excited about it. I'm excited about it. I think we can get Dr. Jeffries into it.

Adding yet another perspective on how these clinical decisions reflect on the body politic, the following is an excerpt from one of the lead investigators on the PLCO trial.[3]

I became the principal investigator at our center for the PLCO study. As you know, it was a multicenter, randomized, prospective controlled trial of screening for three different kinds of cancer including prostate cancer. The techniques that were applied to screen for prostate cancer in men included prostate specific antigen (PSA). We showed no mortality benefit for those who were screened. As you might guess, the publication of our results was met with a great deal of criticism . . . with what I consider to be the biases that are inherent in defending practice patterns that have already been pretty well ensconced in the minds of the physicians who apply them or offer them to their patients. Once a screening tool has already been adopted into practice because there's a strong belief both on the part of the doctors who are administering or ordering the test and patients who are clamoring to have the test done because they don't want to have a delayed diagnosis and die or have morbid complications. So it becomes a little tricky in terms of backing away from use of that screening tool until and if you have solid data upon which you can make conclusions and recommendations that it's either good or it's not good.

Just in the past week or two, the US health services issued a statement in support of the conclusions that we, the PLCO investigators, reached from analyzing our data. Using PSA and digital rectal examinations really doesn't offer benefit to the men who choose to be screened, but the treatment is associated with side effects or complications that are significant. I believe the results of our study, PLCO, do not advocate for that type of screening when given the opportunity to offer my opinion. So in a nutshell that's kind of what we did and what the results were and what my opinion is.

The urologists have told me that they think PSA screening still is the correct way to take care of people and the health of their prostate glands. What we emphasized is the, not only has it not changed the death rate but there are complications associated with going ahead with treatment, when in fact treatment may not be necessary because of the fact that the, you have a – blocking on the words right now – not a lead-time bias, but an overdiagnosis bias, that's what I'm searching for.

I think for many patients the notion that you have a cancer and that you want to do nothing about it and sit tight is anathema. I don't know the data on this, it probably drives an awful lot of the decision-making afterwards because people are just not comfortable that they can live with cancer and not die from the cancer or suffer greatly from the cancer.

Well I don't know what we charge for performing a PSA. I don't know what the dollar figure is at our institution, it's I'm sure comparable to wherever it's done. Let me estimate that it's a $200 test. If you apply that to men over the age of 50 and do so on an annual basis. I can't do the math that quickly here in my head, but we are talking about many millions of dollars just to do the screen. And then the follow-up study, which probably includes repeating the PSA to be sure that there's not a laboratory error here and confirm that it's truly elevated. That adds additional cost. Then there are the doctor's fees for whatever clinical assessment is done. Biopsies often will follow and that jumps the cost a lot more. Followed by a radical prostatectomy and/or radiation therapy treatments. Again, I don't know the cost of doing a radical prostatectomy. I will guess that it's significantly upwards of $50,000 when you add the hospital, the operating room, and the surgeon's fee, pathologist's fee, and so on and so forth. So you've begun to spend a lot of money to do all these different things and you've created incontinence, lack of potency as two of the more significant downstream problems associated with treatment that the patient will then deal with perhaps for the rest of his life. It becomes a tremendously costly phenomenon.

We're beginning to see in the lay literature a little bit more in the way of thoughts about constraining some of the things that we do in our medical practice and asking your doctor. Why does he want to do this and expecting the Dr. to answer the questions that are asked not with defensiveness, but rather with data that support the practice that he's recommending. We're spending 17 percent of the gross domestic product right now on medical care and we are headed upwards of 20 percent in the near future if we don't change some of the things that we're doing. And society collectively is gonna say, "We can't afford that. It's just too much money." And you have to get the members of society to believe that's true in order to change practice patterns. Doctors can't impose this upon society. Everybody has to be in agreement that this is something that we need to do. End-of-life care, for example, should often be switched to a hospice-like approach for the care of those patients rather than continue the aggressiveness in trying to push death away. We can't do that.

And I think that if we as a society and as physicians can't learn how to constrain ourselves, we are going to be limited by governmental controls that are imposed upon our practice, which will affect me as a practitioner, but it will affect my patients too. We have to learn to engage our brains and practice with evidence much more than what we do right now.

This informant talked about Americans not being comfortable with a diagnosis of cancer and not willing to change our cultural model of cancer. Yet, active surveillance could be an ideal standard of care.

This problem is not limited to prostate cancer. Approximately one-third of Medicare expenditures occur in the final year of life and much of that is concentrated in the last month of life, mostly for life-sustaining care. Americans are now spending 17 percent of gross domestic product on healthcare. The healing ritual is a process where individuals engage healers to deal with death or the potential of death. Yet everyone must die. The healing ritual depends on an accurate diagnosis, yet there is a well-established diagnosis within biomedicine that is almost never used: futility. The diagnosis implies the treatment. The appropriate treatment for futility is to stop treatment. There is no moral obligation for physicians to provide healthcare that is futile. Yet it is an extremely difficult diagnosis to make, knowing that persuasion is also a component of diagnosis. Persuasion within a healing relationship is completely different than persuasion for a patient without an established healing relationship. The diagnosis of "the process of dying" is far simpler when the patient has already trusted the doctor in situations where disease and death defined the scope of the social relationship. The existential threat of impending death can be negotiated within a healing relationship – I've done it. Like all diagnoses, an incorrect diagnosis is a catastrophe but an accurate diagnosis provides a necessary social function. It might be that healing relationships, the consequence of the healing ritual, are a necessary but beleaguered cultural component of our healthcare system. This research project is an invitation to my fellow anthropologists to study Western biomedicine as the unmarked category, the cultural performance where for the most part things go well, not the easily observable disasters. Even though the Institute of Medicine (IOM) never explained what a continuous healing relationship actually was, they recognized its importance. Describing the social practices that constitute continuous healing relationships is a task for anthropologists.

Healing relationships articulated by social institutions

Both the Institute of Medicine (IOM) and the National Institutes of Health (NIH) state the underlying hypothesis: healing relationships improve quality of care and outcomes. There is some evidence that this is true (Kelley et al., 2014; Institute 2001; Donaldson et al., 1996; Martin et al., 2007).

American values

The core values of life, liberty, and the pursuit of happiness are foundational in American society. If you overlay those values on federal governmental spending, *life* is represented by Medicare and Medicaid; *liberty* by the Defense Budget; and *the pursuit of happiness* by Social Security retirement. Those three budgetary items constitute approximately 90 percent of government spending. Recall the patient who had damaged genitalia and teared up when discussing his lapse in Medicaid coverage. I commented that his one tear would evoke hundreds of words in an illness narrative. That one tear would probably need millions of words to express America's healthcare policy debates. We are currently deeply divided between healthcare as a fundamental right or healthcare as a commodity that should be regulated by market forces.

Notes

1 http://nordic.cochrane.org/sites/nordic.cochrane.org/files/public/uploads/mammography_screening_leads_to_substantial_overdiagnosis.pdf_letterhead.pdf (accessed February 1, 2017).
2 www.auanet.org/content/media/USPSTF_information_sheet.pdf (accessed January 1, 2013).
3 PLCO trial is one of two prospective randomized prostate screening trials in existence; this one showed no benefit for screening with PSA.

References

Brawley, O. W., and Goldberg, P. 2011. *How We Do Harm: A Doctor Breaks Ranks About Being Sick in America*. New York: St. Martin's Press.

Brownlee, S. 2007. *Overtreated: Why Too Much Medicine Is Making Us Sicker and Poorer*. New York: Bloomsbury.

Carter, S. M., Rogers, W., Degeling, C., Douse, E. J., and Barratt, A. 2015. The Challenge of Overdiagnosis Begins With Its Definition. *BMJ (Online)*: 350.

Donaldson, M. S., Lohr, K. N., and Vaneslow, N. A. (eds.). 1996. *Primary Care: America's Health in a New Era*. Washington, DC: National Academy Press.

Institute of Medicine. 2001. *Crossing the Quality Chasm: A New Health System for the 21st Century*. Washington, DC: National Academy Press.

Kelly, J. M., G. Kraft-Todd, L. Schapira, and J.K.H. Reiss. 2014. The Influence of the Patient-Clinician Relationship on Healthcare Outcomes: A Systematic Review and Meta-Analysis of Randomized Controlled Trials. *PLoS ONE 9*.

Martin, J. C., R. F. Avant, and M. A. Bowmann. 2007. The Future of Family Medicine: A Collaborative Project of the Family Medicine Community. *Annals of Family Medicine*: S3–32.

Meza, J. P. 2015. Screening Mammography Requires Informed Consent. *Clinical Research in Practice: The Journal of Team Hippocrates* 1.

Miller, A. B., C. Wall, C. J. Baines, S. Ping, and T. To. 2014. Twenty-Five Year Follow-Up for Breast Cancer Incidence and Mortality of the Canadian National Breast Screening Study: Randomised Screening Trial. *BMJ*: 348.

Welch, G., Schwartz, L. M., and Woloshin, S. 2011. *Overdiagnosed: Making People Sick in the Pursuit of Health*. Boston: Beacon Press.

Part V
Narrative studies on healing reconsidered

16 Narrative healing reconsidered

Introduction

As a scholar, I find limited value to deconstruct a social process unless the pieces are reassembled into a more useful theoretical construct. In this chapter, I offer my opinion about correctives and challenges to narrative studies related to healing. I see systematic errors that are self-reinforcing and deserve comment. I challenge other anthropologists to critically appraise these topics before using them in their own work.

Regarding others who have written about narrative studies on healing, I believe we agree far more than we disagree and that we can all improve together. One of the most important aspects of this project was to reorganize and synthesize disparate writings into a conceptual whole with a common foundation. Although I point out my disagreements in this chapter, the next chapter reviews aspects of narrative healing that I hope demonstrate a common foundation.

In a substantial review of narrative and anthropology, Cheryl Mattingly and Linda Garro organize chapters originating from the Harvard Friday Morning Seminar in medical anthropology, resulting in *Narrative and the Cultural Construction of Illness and Healing* (2000). The introduction to that book begins, "Narrative is a fundamental human way of giving meaning to experience" (Mattingly and Garro 2000: 1). They quote Rosaldo:

> Telling stories allows narrators to communicate what is significant in their lives, how things matter to them. Narratives offer a powerful way to shape conduct because they have something to say about what gives life meaning, what is inspiring in our lives, and what is dangerous and worth taking risks for.
>
> (Mattingly and Garro 2000: 11; Rosaldo 1986)

They refer to Carrithers and his discussion of plot as it refers to an inner notion of what will happen as well as an outer sense of "landscape" (Carrithers 1992; Mattingly and Garro 2000: 3). Narrative connects storyteller and audience, is a powerful method of socialization, and mediates emergent constructions of reality.

> Stories also concern events as experienced and suffered through by quite specific actors. They allow us (the audience) to infer something about what it feels like to be in that story world, that is, they give form to feeling. Telling the story is a "relational act" that necessarily implies the audience.
>
> (Mattingly and Garro 2000: 11)

I hope my ethnography stimulates reconsideration of who is the audience. Mattingly and Garro also acknowledge the alternate side of the power equation, quoting Ochs and Capps, "Narrative practices, including who is entitled to tell a story and when it can be told, 'reflect an established power relations in a wide-ranging domestic and community institutions'" (Mattingly and Garro 2000: 3; Ochs and Capps 1996). I discuss this further in what follows. Mattingly and Garro summarize these themes as represented in the body of work in anthropology and other disciplines engaged in the study of narrative.

Although I agree with everything they wrote, I find it striking that "the doctor" is left out of a discussion of narrative healing. This is a glaring omission. I hope this ethnography extends the boundaries to include narrative healing that occurs between doctors and patients. My data suggest that doctors tell stories that connect patients as listeners in a relational act that creates an emergent reality and relieves suffering.

In Lawrence Kirmayer's chapter on "broken narratives," he states:

> Patient and clinician are actors engaged in conversation; although they need each other to tell and enact their stories, at the same time they wrestle with each other to see whose version of the story will be lived. This wrestling itself may become part of the final version of the story, or it may be suppressed to construct an authorizing genealogy. Once authorized and accepted, the story is retold and so persists, becomes stabilized, and influences future stories.
>
> (Kirmayer 2000: 156)

Kirmayer uses the word "wrestle," and differing versions of the story "compete" to become realized and a reality that is retold. He later says, "These situations of conflict and contestation can reveal structural problems and ideological conflicts in medical care; at the same time, they provide important opportunities for the creation of new meaning" (Kirmayer 2000: 157). I fundamentally disagree with the portrayal of healing as a contest between the patient and clinician. In a contest, there are winners and losers. This ethnography is an effort to move past those notions. The patients and doctors I observed enjoyed genuine relationships of intimacy creating a "win-win" scenario (Covey 1989). I espouse relationship-centered care (Beach and Inui

2006), which adequately addresses the moral overtones so often invoked by narrativists writing about healing.

In the final chapter, "Emergent Narratives," Mattingly asks,

> What has any of this to do with healing? What can we see about healing if we discover narrative moments, times when healing and recovery take on all the compelling power of the well-told story? It may bring us closer to the perspective of the sufferer.
>
> (Mattingly 2000: 206)

In this excerpt, the perspective of the sufferer is metonymically correlated with healing. Absent again is the doctor or healer. More importantly, the cultural context of healing is absent. She summarizes by saying,

> This evangelical bent, this need to act as transformative agents and not as mere technicians of the body, drives even some Western healers to engage in the creation of healing dramas in their efforts to assist clients in transforming their lives.
>
> (Mattingly 2000: 207)

Note the implied critique of biomedicine as "mere technicians" and the implied rarity of "even some" Western healers engage in healing. I contend that Mattingly overlooked the biggest healing drama of all – existential threats, the diagnosis narrative, and the healing ritual story. Western biomedicine does engage in healing – through creating a story that matters to the patient with the reportability of responding to an existential threat that legitimates a claim on society's resources.

Returning to the preceding quote by Kirmayer, he states, "Once authorized and accepted, the story is retold and so persists, becomes stabilized, and influences future stories." I think that is what has happened to narrative studies related to healing. There has been a "piling on" phenomenon; many assume doctors "dehumanize" suffering patients. This has now become dogma and many narrative writers retell the same version with minimal variation (Engel et al. 2008). "If you repeat it enough, people will think it is true" (linguistic artifact, difficult to attribute accurately).

I contend that the relationship between diagnosis narratives and illness narratives is profoundly misunderstood. They are not by definition in conflict with each other as is so often suggested. I believe they are complementary to each other. I try to explain this complementarity in the following chapters. Suffering exists, but doctors do not cause it – it is the human condition.

Arthur Frank

Arthur Frank writes in the genre of the wounded storyteller, firmly grounded in the world of medicine as a subculture. He describes his book as theoretical but also bases it on his own personal story of undergoing cancer treatment, supplemented with stories from others. He points out, rather dramatically, "Sooner or later, everyone is a wounded storyteller" (Frank 1995: xiii). All of us must at some time face disease or death.

Consistent with the development of narrative in the preceding theoretical considerations, he states, "These embodied stories have two sides, one personal and the other social" (Frank 1995: 2).

> The ill body's articulation in stories is a personal task, but the stories told by the ill are also social. The obvious social aspect of stories is that they are told to someone, whether that person is immediately present or not.
>
> (Frank 1995: 3)

He describes exactly how a schema for storytelling occurs, stating,

> The shape of the telling is molded by all the rhetorical expectations that the storyteller has been internalizing ever since he first heard some relative describe an illness, or she saw her first television commercial for a nonprescription remedy, or he was instructed to "tell the doctor what hurts" and had to figure out what counted as a story that the doctor wanted to hear.
>
> (Frank 1995: 3)

He goes on to say illness stories become a circulation of stories and recounts how he told his personal illness story multiple different times to different people in the course of one day. The stories he described were told while he was in a clinical care context. He goes on to say, "The story of illness that trumps all others in the modern period is the medical narrative. The story told by the physician becomes the one against which others are ultimately judged true or false, useful or not" (Frank 1995: 5). When people accept this authorized medical story, Frank refers to it as "narrative surrender" (Frank 1995: 6). This narrative surrender takes on huge proportion as he goes on to describe its ultimate effect as "medical colonization." In this way, he is describing the control of the body and equating it with control of the story. Arthur Frank's rambling stories about his personal illness lack the rigor of an autoethnography and his book lacks actual data, yet other narrativists almost universally cite him as authoritative. Yet, this often cited text has the scientific standing of an essay. I encourage my colleagues to critically appraise this text in light of the data in this ethnography.

The self can compare and accept or reject a self-narrative, as noted by Tomasello (Tomasello 1999: 52). Frank also echoes Tomasello's sentiments: "The self is understood as coming to be human in relation to others, and the self can only continue to be human by living for the Other" (Frank 1995:

15). Frank acknowledges "the storyteller" and the narrative development of the self. His focus seems to be on who controls the narrative.

My critique of Arthur Frank is that he got it wrong when he chooses "narrative surrender" as the hallmark of a clinical encounter in Western biomedicine; he artificially creates winners and losers, and he portrays the doctor as the antagonist rather than a participant with the narrating self in a struggle with disease and death. Purely on the basis of theoretic musings, I believe that professionals – doctors – can give power to individuals through ritual without diminishing their own cultural power, which seems to me to be a deeply embedded social narrative. I believe that the power is only "borrowed" by the doctor and it is renewable because the locus of power is in the sociocultural domain. Both doctors and patients draw upon the clinical encounter as a cultural practice to perform transformation that benefits both the individual and the culture. I realize this is a discursive maneuver, curtailing discussions of power by redirecting such discussions into the framework of "learning through the other" and narrative transformation. I share musings simply to generate questions as I explore how theorists inform my research.

Frank discusses the work of Arthur and Joan Kleinman in his discussion of the body in medical anthropology (Frank 1995: 28; Kleinman and Kleinman 1994). He uses their term of the "body-self," echoing Scheper-Hughes and Lock's "individual body-self" (Scheper-Hughes and Lock 1987), stating,

> The Kleinmans provide one of the most sophisticated analysis of the interweaving of bodies, cultures, and lives, and the limitations of their efforts to hear the body speaking reveal the dilemma that every such attempt, including my own, must struggle with.
>
> (Frank 1995: 28)

This body-self is actually one side of the triangulated terminology of narrative-embodiment, narrative-self, and body-self. Working with a related term called "self-stories," Frank aggregates all of these terms into a "body-self-story" (Frank 1995: 57). I'm not sure how much more helpful this is other than to point out the metonymic importance of each component.

Claiming that illness is a call for stories, "Stories have to repair the damage that illness is done to the ill person's sense of where she is in life, and where she may be going. Stories are a way of redrawing maps and finding new destinations" (Frank 1995: 53). Again, I caution about the conflation of terminology that I believe has left this area of inquiry dense. I contend it is not illness, but disease, that forms the call for stories. Additionally, it is the self – not the person – that must self-narrate the story. Here again I differentiate the duality of illness/person as contrasted to disease/self as vital concepts to understand healing rituals as social practice and healing relationships as two selves recognizing each other as being like the other and being capable of entering into an authentic relationship.

Frank quotes Schafer:

> In telling the self-stories to others we may, for most purposes, be said to be performing straightforward narrative actions. In saying that we also tell them to ourselves, however, we are enclosing one story within another. This is a story that there is a self to tell something to, a someone else serving as audience who is oneself or one's self . . . On this view, the self is a telling.
>
> (Frank 1995: 55–56)

The process of telling a story reaffirms both the relationships with others and the self. Elaborating further, he says,

> We need to tell someone else a story that describes our experience because the process of creating a story also creates the memory structure that will contain the gist of the story for the rest of our lives. Talking is remembering. Memory is not only restored in the illness story; more significantly, memory is created. If the story being told . . . something to live up to, then a future is also being created, and that future carries a distinct responsibility.
>
> (Frank 1995: 61)

When Frank reverts to the self as narrator, I concur with his description. Notice the congruence with D'Andrade's term "narrative schema" and the preceding description. The "future" is the relationship between objects that are expected, given the particular narrative schema deployed. Tomasello would describe it as intentionality.

Throughout the rest of the book Frank outlines a taxonomy for three different illness story schemas: the restitution narrative, the chaos narrative, and the quest narrative. He characterizes the restitution narrative as "surrendering one's body to the medical world . . . the high-tech medical world remains a perpetual source of the hope that keeps restitution stories going" (Frank 1995: 174). Frank's word choice of "surrender" reveals a judgmental perspective. "Surrendering to the restitution narrative" (losing the preferred self) is somehow construed as the unmarked category, the norm. My research challenges that perspective.

Although Arthur Frank described a heuristic to classify narratives, Andrew Sparkes and Brett Smith provide ethnographic data in their article, "When Narratives Matter: Men, Sport, and Spinal Cord Injuries" (2006). They use Frank's taxonomy of illness stories (restitution, chaos, and quest narratives), but provide actual examples from patients with spinal cord injury. The authors sort their ethnographic data using this taxonomy, reinforcing Frank's heuristic (Sparkes and Smith 2006). Their work is interesting in that they describe the same patient population that Cheryl Mattingly studied. It is Mattingly's work, not Arthur Frank's, that I used as an embarkation for my research. Perhaps it is my pragmatism, but Frank's heuristic adds no value when confronted with actual suffering patients dealing with existential threats. The danger of course is that we understand healing even less.

Byron J. Good and Mary-Jo DelVecchio Good

Mattingly's comment about doctors' "anti-narrative speech" (Mattingly 1998: 12) has adherents in the writings of Byron J. Good and Mary-Jo DelVecchio Good (Good and Good 2000). I believe this attitude prevents further investigation into healing relationships. If anthropologists uniformly expect to see abuse of power, then the observation bias created by this analytical lens cripples the ability of anthropologists to see other aspects of the clinical encounter between patients and doctors, an example of inattentional blindness (Simmons and Chabris 1999). This is particularly important for a discipline that relies so heavily on participant observation and in an area of research that has gotten so little attention – actual ethnographic data of Western biomedical clinical encounters with doctors. I observed intimate, trusting relationships between doctors and patients where each knows personal details of the other. These authentic relationships never came at the beginning of the healing ritual – they only occurred after the ritual healing was complete. There is no power differential in an authentic relationship – both are vulnerable and known to each other. I believe that the healing relationship is a form of *communitas* between the doctor and the patient – a social relationship that occurs at the completion of a ritual. I believe it is inaccurate for anthropologists to continue to "pile on" and continue to portray doctors as abusing social authority in a generalized way. What exists in the anthropological canon is a rich description of the marked category of bad doctoring. Of course there are bad doctors – patients tell those experiences as horror stories. I fully acknowledge these experiences occur, but they are not the majority. The unmarked category – when doctors provide relief and help patients – is far more common but not well recorded in the ethnographic record related to narrative healing.

Byron Good and Mary-Jo DelVecchio Good discuss narrative in the medical setting. The following statement repeats a common critique of Western biomedicine:

> In spite of the ubiquity of storytelling in medical settings or in research with healthcare practitioners, one prominent form of critique of medical care has been based on physicians' failure to recognize the narrative dimensions of the illness experience, to attend to the stories the patients tell. Physicians constitute "disease" as disordered physiological structure and function, set within abstract, medicalized time, or as "dehistorisized objects-in-themselves." Thus while patients experience "sickness" in the context of life narratives, the lived body, and diverse forms of social relations and power structures, medicine constructs the

objects of therapeutic attention as ahistorical, atemporal, and nonsocial dimensions of the medicalized body.

(Good and Good 2000: 51)

This type of statement sets the general frame of medical anthropology as a critique of biomedicine. Here, the Goods are repeating Arthur Kleinman's critique of Western medicine, demonstrating the generalized acceptance of this perspective within the corpus of work in narrative and healing. I contest this perspective as incomplete based on my discussion of clinical encounter as a healing ritual. Healing rituals are very engaged with self-stories, are set in a temporal context of a life span, and are social performances, all attributes contradictory to the statement by Good and DelVecchio Good. Further emphasizing their point, Good and DelVecchio Good go on to repeat the metaphor of the colonized dimension of the medical lifeworld. They state:

Stories such as these [reflective stories] complement the formalized medical stories of the wards, revealing aspects of the inner life of medicine and serving in a modest way to protest against dehumanizing aspects of ward culture. Seldom, however, do they lead to serious efforts to change the structure of clinical life. Even more seldom do they lead to any serious questioning of the basic structure the narrative practices through which disease is constituted as the object of medical attention.

(Good and Good 2000: 65)

In a rather damning commentary, they label this dichotomy as a *moral failure* (Good and Good 2000: 62). I find that comment un-anthropological; such disciplinary ethnocentrism is synonymous with "not valid." They claim a "story" told to an anthropologist has more validity than actual observation. In fact, I believe this is exactly where the sampling bias of emphasizing the "marked" category in most narrative healing scholarship originates. It simply does not fit with my data, which I have previously stated tries to correct a biased sampling error in the extant ethnographic record. Having observed very similar medical education encounters, I have a much more anthropological perspective, seeing the distress of medical learners as a rite of passage (Meza and Provenzano 2015).

Cheryl Mattingly

Although I admire the work of Cheryl Mattingly more than others, she also joins this bias in anthropological narrative healing literature. Yet, she, like many, portrays the doctor as the antagonist, such as when she summarizes the anthropological canon, saying:

Narrative studies of patient/doctor communication have addressed power through examination of a subordinate (patient) voice which is in contest with a prevailing and powerful medical voice. Analysis of interchanges between doctors and their patients often show patient narratives as neglected or reorganized through the doctor's "medicalizing" discussion. . . . "Doctor talk" often emerges as a kind of anti-narrative speech act, a "literary rhetoric," which gains its perlocutionary power precisely through a set of discursive moves which suppress personal narrative, such as adoption of the passive voice and consequent elimination of agency.

(Mattingly 1998: 12)

In this characterization, Mattingly reinforces the concept that doctors medicalize and therefore subordinate patient voice in an anti-narrative rhetoric, which implies an abuse of power. I believe this portrayal is a widespread critical flaw in narrative healing studies. Doctors only have power because of cultural authority in their role as healers. I have made an argument that Western biomedicine follows the same healing ritual as cultures throughout time and around the globe. So why do we as anthropologists consider Western biomedicine worthy of being singled out for judgment as a form of oppression? It is much more logical to view both the patient and the doctor participating in a common culture. In the theoretical frame of this book, I gave an alternate version of the relationship between the self and society; the relationship between the self and society reframes this oft-repeated trope about doctors "medicalizing" patients. If we consider the diagnosis narrative as an integral part of a healing ritual story that brings relief to the suffering patient, then the individual has access to a completely new illness story through participation in this socially authorized practice.

Again, Mattingly acknowledges anthropology's excessive critique of biomedicine and then almost immediately finds a new way to relegate biomedical practitioners to the role of "bad guy":

We [anthropologists] have documented the miscommunications which so often characterize patients' discussions with doctors and other healers of Western medicine. We have also criticized the culture of biomedicine for being insufficiently mindful of personal, familial, institutional and cultural factors that influence how a disabling condition is experienced and handled by the person who is ill. We have been less attentive to how the illness experience is addressed in clinical practice, especially among lower-status health professionals who spend sustained time with patients. A hospital world operates in two time spaces. One is the time paradigmatically expressed by the doctor – fast and efficient. Doctors cannot afford to linger too long in any one spot. The other is the time of the lesser health professional: therapists, aides, sometimes nurses. Things move more slowly here. These professionals may spend an hour or more a day with a patient, and some of this may be quite informal.

(Mattingly 1998: 21)

Mattingly presents no data whatsoever of how doctors interact with patients but relegates them to "fast time," implying insufficient time to address real concerns. My data show that doctors often spend an hour and a half talking with patients and families in the office setting, hours interacting with multiple institutions, to be able to perform surgeries that often take two to four hours to perform. That is not "fast time." Mattingly then sets up the false dichotomy of the doctors versus "the lesser health professionals," valorizing their sacrifice of time and effort. This dichotomy reveals systematic bias that prevents anthropologists from observing what really happens between a doctor and a patient. When I read Mattingly's comments about "doctor time," I was struck by the distorted, pejorative description. I personally did medical consultations in a rehabilitation unit for over a decade. I saw occupational therapists treating three or more patients simultaneously, billing each patient as if they were getting individualized therapy. I did review the medical concerns quickly – blood pressure, vital signs, blood sugar, medication review, and so forth. During those visits, the occupational therapist billed and was compensated far more than I, the doctor. I also remember in one of those quick encounters I diagnosed a life-threatening condition – a pulmonary embolism. This was an existential threat where the patient might not survive another 24 hours. There in the rehabilitation unit I spent half a day ordering diagnostic tests and transferring the patient to a medical-surgical bed to initiate therapy. The occupational therapist would wander over and wrote progress notes, "Too unstable – will follow." The occupational therapist used "fast time" when the context changed. When Mattingly wrote "doctor time" she was devaluing that interaction and implying the work of the occupational therapist was more important. Given the differing existential threat, the doctor and therapist had different healing roles. That patient saw me for years afterwards and always said, "You're the doctor that saved my life." He never discussed his occupational therapy sessions.

Instead of repeating these claims, I suggest we recognize this as a sampling error. Mattingly's comments about "doctor time" are only true in an inpatient rehabilitation setting. This ethnography contradicts Mattingly's generalization to clinical encounters in the office or late at night after everyone has left the hospital – a time to go back and spend a human moment with someone you operated on the day before.

I understand that it is far easier to criticize a work than to produce the work initially. I wrote this ethnography as a corrective to theoretical inadequacies in anthropology. I see a different perspective that opens new avenues to narrative healing and medical anthropology research. Extant theoretical framings were inadequate to explain my data. I turn next to positioning my work within the context of the work of Cheryl Mattingly and Arthur Kleinman. I understand that I am standing on the shoulders of giants.

References

Beach, Mary Catherine, and Thomas Inui. 2006. Relationship-Centered Care – A Constructive Reframing. *Journal of General Internal Medicine* 21:S3–S8.

Carrithers, Michael. 1992. *Why Humans Have Cultures*. Oxford: Oxford University Press.

Covey, Stephen R. 1989. *The 7 Habits of Highly Effective People*. New York: Free Press.

Engel, John D., et al. 2008. *Narrative in Health Care: Healing Patients, Practitioners, Profession, and Community*. Oxford: Radcliffe.

Frank, Arthur W. 1995. *The Wounded Storyteller: Body, Illness, and Ethics*. Chicago: University of Chicago Press.

Good, Byron J., and Mary-Jo DelVecchio Good. 2000. "Fiction" and "Historicity" in Doctors' Stories: Social and Narrative Dimensions of Learning Medicine. *In Narrative and the Cultural Construction of Illness and Healing*. C. Mattingly and L. C. Garro, eds. Pp. 50–69. Berkeley: University of California Press.

Kirmayer, Laurence. 2000. Broken Narratives: Clinical Encounters and the Poetics of Illness Experience. *In Narrative and the Cultural Construction of Illness and Healing*. C. Mattingly and L. Garro, eds. Berkeley: University of California Press.

Kleinman, Arthur, and Joan Kleinman. 1994. How Bodies Remember: Social Memory and Bodily Experience of Criticism, Resistance, and Delegitimation Following China's Cultural Revolution. *New Literary History* 25:710–711.

Mattingly, Cheryl. 1998. *Healing Dramas and Clinical Plots: The Narrative Structure of Experience*. Cambridge: Cambridge University Press.

———. 2000. Emergent Narratives. *In Narrative and the Cultural Construction of Illness and Healing*. C. Mattingly and L. C. Garro, eds. Pp. 181–211. Berkeley: University of California Press.

Mattingly, Cheryl, and Linda C. Garro, eds. 2000. *Narrative and the Cultural Construction of Illness and Healing*. Berkeley: University of California Press.

Meza, James P., and Anthony Provenzano. 2015. Understanding Pimping as a Rite of Passage: An Enduring Cultural Practice in Medical Education. *MedEdPublish* 4:9.

Ochs, Elinor, and Lisa Capps. 1996. Narrating the Self. *Annual Review of Anthropology* 25:19–43.

Rosaldo, Renato. 1986. Ilongot Hunting as Story and Experience. *In The Anthropology of Experience*. V. M. Turner and E. N. Bruner, eds. Urbana: University of Illinois Press.

Scheper-Hughes, N., and M. M. Lock. 1987. The Mindful Body: A Prolegomenon to Future Work in Medical Anthropology. *Medical Anthropology Quarterly* 1:6–41.

Simmons, Daniel, and Christopher Chabris. 1999. Gorillas in Our Midst: Sustained Inattentional Blindness for Dynamic Events. *Perception* 28:1059–1074.

Sparkes, Andrew C., and Brett M. Smith. 2006. When Narratives Matter: Men, Sport, and Spine Cord Injury. *In The Self in Health and Illness: Patients, Professionals and Narrative Identity*. F. Rapport and P. Wainwright, eds. Pp. 53–68. Oxford: Radcliffe.

Tomasello, Michael. 1999. *The Cultural Origins of Human Cognition*. Cambridge, MA: Harvard University Press.

17 Theoretical synthesis

Ethnography advances theory. While narrative theory is ubiquitous, I want to focus on how narrative relates to healing. Having struggled with my data and the anthropological canon on the topic, I plan to demonstrate the logical consistencies and common foundation my work shares with two of the most prominent writers in the field. Additionally, I want to share an analytical frame that combines them into a consistent whole – a new model for inquiry and education.

Cheryl Mattingly

Of all the anthropologists writing in the field of narrative healing, I admire Cheryl Mattingly the most. I have read her book *Healing Dramas and Clinical Plots: The Narrative Structure of Experience* at least a dozen times. I believe her arguments about narrative and experience are breakthrough theoretical discoveries, which explains why I emphasized them in this analysis. I would not have been able to write this book had I not used her work as a foundation. She herself sees her work as a point of departure from previous works in narrative healing.

Cheryl Mattingly's aforementioned work approaches my own understanding of healing practices most closely. Mattingly effectively develops the argument that narrative structure, experience, and ritual converge to produce healing dramas. She recognizes the contribution of cognitive anthropology to narrative, acknowledges that narrative exists prior to experience, discusses time in narrative as well as ritual time, and argues for therapeutic emplotment as a model of healing practice. Emplotment, as used by Mattingly, is a form of experiential therapy sessions that use an emergent structure. I endorse her metonymic use of narration and experience as co-constituent – each begets the other. Recall Jerome Bruner in the theoretical section of this book described this same concept. Mattingly also invokes Edith Turner:

> Narratives become one medium through which the healer tries to connect a person's individual experience to an ideal or preferred narrative,

and healing itself is equated with the rhetorical task of persuading the patient to see her experience in a certain way (Turner 1992). Stories which are located in ritual actions may take on special therapeutic powers; indeed, certain kinds of stories may have their special place as an integral part of a healing ritual.

(Mattingly 1998: 14)

She acknowledges the transformative properties of healing, and challenges the dominant assumption that the primary purpose of narrative is to give the self a sense of coherence.

Mattingly suggests that the necessary precursor to therapeutic emplotment is "locating desire" in a social drama and arises by the work of the therapist in creating multiple possible imagined endings to the narrative drama. Because Mattingly studied occupational therapists, she missed the importance of diagnosis narratives in healing-ritual narratives. Only doctors or leeches make socially authorized diagnoses. I contend that W.H.R. Rivers correctly identified how an "existential threat" creates the "universal desire" to enter into healing rituals with doctors or therapists. I understand Mattingly's terminology, "locating desires," as the client's future experiences which are existentially threatened by disability and the therapist is actually proposing treatment plans to deal with future threats to "the story" from a newly limited set of possibilities.

Critically appraising Mattingly's ethnography of healing dramas, I realized she includes hardly any illness narratives in her own data. In that way, her data is similar to my own. No one comments on its absence, but I believe that the reason for her lack of attention to illness narratives is the same as the reason my dataset lacks illness narratives; we were both looking at ritual as narratively structured experience. She and I both focus on activities that the practitioner and patient do together using observational methods. Mattingly defines narrative in a way that also offers a privileged perspective on the lived experiences of patients, not one told to an anthropologist but one experienced in the presence of the anthropologist. She gives the "experience-near" account that anthropologists strive for, the emic experience:

To summarize, three features of narrative form make it especially appropriate for addressing illness and healing experiences. One, narratives are event-centered. They concern action, more specifically human action, even more specifically, human interaction. They concern social actions. Two, narratives are experience-centered. They do not merely describe what someone does in the world but what the world does to that someone. They allow us to infer something about what it feels like to be in that story world. Narratives also recount those events that happen unwilled, unpredicted, and often unwished for by the actors, even if those very actors set the events in motion in the first place. Narratives, one could say, are about the unintended consequences of action (Arendt 1958). Three, narratives do not merely refer to past experience but create experiences for their audience. Narratives mean to be provocative. They request a different response from the audience than denotative prose. Narrative offers meaning through evocation, image, the mystery of the unsaid. It persuades by seducing the listener into the world it portrays, unfolding events in a suspense-laden time in which one wonders what will happen next.

(Mattingly 1998: 9)

Mattingly contrasts her experiential narrative (narrative as ritual) and highlights the difference between narratives as "experience" versus narrative as "denotative prose" (illness narratives).

Mattingly says,

> That is, therapists and patients not only tell stories, sometimes they create story-like structures through their interactions. Furthermore, this effort at story-making, which I will refer to as therapeutic emplotment, is integral to the healing power of this practice. Thus, this book considers the narrative structure of action and experience.
>
> (Mattingly 1998: 2)

Again, using my own data, I could very well have written the same sentence. "Doctors and patients not only tell stories, they create story-like structures through their interactions. Furthermore, this story making activity, which I refer to as the healing ritual, is integral to the healing power of this practice."

Although her entire ethnography is based on an exploration of narrative theory, Mattingly portrays the therapist-client interaction as a healing ritual. This portrayal of narrative as ritual is foundational to my research. Mattingly joins other anthropologists in understanding the transformative powers of ritual and ritual narrative:

> Healers may draw upon narrative to encourage powerful reframings of illness that actively change the sufferer's perception of his own body and personal experience. In studies of healing rituals, narratives (often cultural myths) are treated as one among a range of multi-media poetic forms that give ritual it perlocutionary power (Leach 1976; Tambiah 1977). Narratives become one medium through which the healer tries to connect a person's individual experience to an ideal or preferred narrative, and healing itself is equated with the rhetorical task of persuading the patient to see her experience in a certain way (Turner 1992). Stories which are located in ritual actions may take on special therapeutic

powers; indeed, certain kinds of stories may have their special place as an integral part of a healing ritual.

(Mattingly 1998: 14)

I use this text to frame the entire argument for my research.

Mattingly recognizes and describes such a narratively informed ritual, complete with narrative persuasion to a preferred narrative to produce the therapeutic transformation. This is why I say that Mattingly most closely approximates my model of healing. She incorporates ritual, persuasion to a preferred narrative, and reframing or transformations of the self-story. Her data and interpretation do not emphasize the illness narrative in any substantial way. As we both focus on ritual aspects of healing, the historical illness narrative is not the experience that creates a healing narrative; it is the narrative structure of the therapeutic experience (ritual) on which both Mattingly and I focus our analysis.

Although Mattingly joins the chorus critiquing biomedicine, her actual data and theoretical framework are consistent with my work. Because of the homologous foundational concepts she uses are identical to the ones I purport in my data, I conclude that we actually described the same social process. We differ in only one exception: Mattingly focused on an existential threat in the potential future and I focused on the existential threat of disease in the present. This common structure of ritual healing accommodates both Mattingly's data and my own. I want to emphasize this commonality and suggest a summative perspective on healing. I explore next another part of healing rituals that I believe are part of the bigger theoretical perspective.

Arthur Kleinman

Both Arthur Kleinman and I agree on the basic premise that enhancing healing in medical practice will improve the healthcare system and patient outcomes. This is the identical argument made by Rita Charon (2006). I completely agree with Arthur Kleinman's description of the role of the doctor (Kleinman 2014). I recently had the privilege of hearing him speak at Harvard Medical School, and his intellect, social analysis, and insight are impressive.[1] Kleinman's seminal text *Illness Narratives: Suffering, Healing, and the Human Condition* created a paradigm. Singularly, that book sparked the "narrative turn" in healing studies by anthropologists. Textual artifacts remain throughout the anthropological literature and medical education referencing that book written in 1988. Illness narratives themselves endure almost unchanged from his definition arising from that text.

Because I want to demonstrate the common theoretical foundations, I will use that text to embark on how my work relates to his. We used vastly different methodologies and approached the topic from completely different levels of analysis. I believe the difference in methodology and level of analysis explains why our findings and conclusions diverge. Comparing methodologies facilitates an understanding how illness narratives and diagnosis narratives exist simultaneously in different places and social contexts. Kleinman set out to study the relationship between medicine, psychiatry, and culture. In *Patients and Healers in the Context of Culture: An Exploration of the Borderland Between Anthropology, Medicine, and Psychiatry*, Kleinman writes:

> The reader will find this book contains a dialectical tension between two reciprocally related orientations: it is both a cross-cultural (largely anthropological) perspective on the essential components of clinical care and a clinical perspective on anthropological studies of medicine and psychiatry. That dialectic is embodied in my own academic training and professional life, so that this book is a personal statement.
>
> (Kleinman 1980: ix)

This work relies almost exclusively on cross-cultural ethnographic data collected in Taiwan and incorporates multiple different ethnomedicine perspectives. Upon closer examination of his ethnographic data, he studied patients with psychiatric distress presenting to psychiatric clinics. He argues (successfully) that illness experiences and broader culture are related. It is in this book that he presents most of his primary ethnographic data. In his *Illness Narratives* (Kleinman 1988), he repeats the argument for a broader audience, using his American clinical practice and presenting a case series to make the same argument.

Using my positionality as a primary care doctor, I see both psychiatric patients and biomedical patients within the same clinical office setting. I find it imperative to distinguish what the patient needs the most: joint attention to an illness narrative as a reflection of unresolved psychosocial distress from past experiences or joint attention to a biomedical diagnosis narrative of disease in the present. Of course, it is never all of one and none of the other. Kleinman correctly points out that trying to force a biomedical diagnosis as the explanation for unresolved psychosocial distress doesn't work. But, the anthropological canon on healing omits the complementary mismatch – some of the most dissatisfied patients result from a missed or incorrect biomedical diagnosis.

Kleinman's willingness to merge the domains of anthropology, medicine, and psychiatry meant that we had divergent perspectives as part of our respective methodologies. For example, in *The Illness Narratives* Kleinman states:

> From a psychiatric standpoint Alice Alcott was deeply distressed and depressed in response to her chronic illness, but although she was desperate, her state did not warrant the clinical diagnosis of major depressive disorder or any other serious psychiatric syndrome . . . Early in

psychotherapy, our sessions centered on grief for her multiple losses. But as her spirits lifted, she returned to her characteristic denial. The last few times we met, she would discuss her children's problems, her parents' problems, anything but her own.

(Kleinman 1988: 38)

Kleinman presents his case series and follows each case with a section labeled "interpretation." It is in his psychiatric interpretation that he attempts to provide the cultural context and "meaning." Whether he presents these interpretations as anthropologist or as psychiatrist is not clear – both use symbolic thought. Because he is trying to argue that they are co-constituent of each other, it probably did not matter to him. I understand why and how he is trying to put forth his argument, but I also recognize that he opens himself to threats to validity of his analysis by taking this approach. The objectivity and reflexivity required to perform ethnography is not possible when you are also the treating physician – the reader never knows whether you are speaking as the doctor or the anthropologist. Kleinman is clear that he is willing to accept this limitation when he says, "That dialectic is embodied in my own academic training and professional life, so that this book is a personal statement." I find it ironic that the seminal text on illness narratives, Kleinman subordinates the "voice" of the patient by presenting the data using his role as psychiatrist. He chose this trade-off to make his larger point about the connection of illness narratives and culture. Psychiatry reviews experiences in the patient's past to offer clues into current behavior. *I believe that attending to an illness narrative is a method of taking the patient's experience of the past and converting it, through joint attention, to a shared experience in the present for both patient and physician.*

Because I am arguing for a synthetic theoretical perspective, I believe "illness narratives" are the equivalent of a diagnostic narrative when the existential threat occurred in the patient's past experience and was not adequately resolved. I contend the existential threat that occurred in the past and persists in current behaviors is a necessary condition before illness narratives claim ritual power. Existential threats evoke a call for a healer. When that threat is in the past, the doctor was not there and was unable to share the experience. The doctor attending to the patient's illness narrative initiates the healing ritual because it is a way to create a shared experience in the present. My critique of Kleinman is that he overreached in his conclusion. He said that to improve "healing," doctors have to incorporate patients' illness narratives into *every* encounter of biomedical practice. However, the temporality of the existential threat determines the type of ritual performance most appropriate. Kleinman made a huge impact in narrative healing studies in anthropology and almost no impact on medical education and medical practice. I find this regrettable. There is a place for doctors to attend to empathic witnessing of the existential experience (suffering) in the patient's past. By overreaching his claim to all of biomedicine, he ran afoul of institutional power (Bourdieu and Passeron 1990 [1970]) in medical education and clinical practice.

Arthur Kleinman acknowledges that healing rituals are part of Western medicine but considers them flawed by lack of attention to the illness narrative. Consider his frame of reference:

> From an anthropological point of view, recording the case is an example of a secular ritual: it formally replicates a social reality in standardized format to a central problem in the human condition. Like religious rituals, secular rituals express and manipulate key symbols that connect a shared set of values and beliefs to practical action. By observing in this light the writing of a case into the medical record, we should be able to see more clearly the influence of professional values (and the professional's personal preferences) in the care of the chronically ill. To accomplish this end, I will first provide a transcript of a doctor-patient interview and then describe the wording of the physician's formal write-up in the patient's record. I don't contend that the following example is representative; indeed I believe that the degree of professional insensitivity it depicts is unusual. But I do think that the physician's overriding interest in disease and disregard of illness is, regrettably, commonplace.
>
> (Kleinman 1988: 131)

The lack of attention to the illness narrative in the healing ritual is "regrettable" for Kleinman. Again, this highlights an implied criticism that I contend is unjustified. He concludes that if biomedicine is to become a healing social practice, it must pay more attention to illness narratives. Kleinman says, "This alternative approach [to biomedical practice] originates in the reconceptualization of medical care as (1) empathic witnessing of the existential experience of suffering" (Kleinman 1988: 226). Note that these quotes from Kleinman acknowledge both "ritual" and "existential" aspects of chronic illness. This shared foundation leads me to believe we agree on healing practices. Problems occur when doctors try to diagnose a biomedical problem as a manifestation of current disease when in fact, the existential threat occurred in the past and the current symptoms refer to an experience in the patient's past. *If we carefully differentiate the temporal locus of the existential threat, then the correct therapy will be structured by the ritual structure described by Kleinman, myself, or Mattingly. All three of us claim that healing occurs through a ritually structured social process that allows for shared experience between the healer and patient.*

Upon reviewing each of Kleinman's cases – Alice Scott, Howard Harris, Rudolph Kristiva, Antigone Paget, William Steele, Patrick Esposito, Paul Sensabaugh, and so forth – I find that Kleinman picked diagnostic "narrative failures" instead of the success stories of biomedicine. In both *Patients and Healers in the Context of Culture* (1980) and *The Illness Narratives*

(1988) Kleinman uses cases that present to psychiatric clinics or consultations. I suggest that there is an inherent selection bias in studying only this population. From each of these cases, he recorded an illness narrative and, based on his psychiatric interpretation, suggested a "healing narrative." He explains this:

> I see medical psychotherapy, then, as a collaborative relationship within which the techniques for exploring illness meanings encourage catharsis, persuasion, practical problem solving, and other of the mechanisms of psychotherapeutic change. . . . When the tasks of support, attention to emotional needs, the negotiation of an authentic relationship are accomplished in a caring fashion the question of how to do medial psychotherapy vanishes. That is the psychotherapy.
>
> (Kleinman 1988: 246)

Kleinman's mistake was to generalize the narrative failures of the diagnosis narrative to all clinical encounters. I am trying to highlight the distinction of illness narratives, as told by a person in a Labovian recall of past experience with diagnosis narratives, which responds to an undifferentiated state of current experience. Both create healing relationships, as experienced by a self, a self completed by interaction with culture, the culture of a medical encounter.

In the introduction to *The Illness Narratives*, Arthur Kleinman (1988) repeats the dominant viewpoint:

> For members of Western societies the body is a discrete entity, a thing, an "it," machine-like and objective, separate from thought and emotion. For members of many non-Western societies, the body is an open system linking social relations to the self, a vital balance between the interrelated elements in the holistic cosmos. Emotion and cognition are integrated into bodily processes. The body – self is not a secularized private domain of the *individual person* [emphasis added] but an organic part of the sacred, socio-centric world, a communicative system involving exchanges with others (including the divine).
>
> (Kleinman 1988: 11)

Instead of using the term individual self he uses the term "individual person" and thereby conflates the theoretical narrator with the cultural construction of the person. Yet, when I re-read this passage, I find that Kleinman's viewpoint is actually true if Western medicine is viewed as a culturally sanctioned ritual, which is my claim. Personhood is a fascinating and valid pursuit of anthropological inquiry; it is just not part of my research project.

Kleinman is consistent with other anthropologists in pointing out that Western civilization emphasizes the individual more than non-Western societies, but he then critiques biomedicine for not legitimating that same individual's unique illness experience. That is inherently contradictory; I emphasize the universality of healing rituals.

One aspect of Kleinman's statement will trump all others. An "authentic relationship" is the marker of a healing relationship. The method by which patients and doctors arrive at an "authentic relationship," a sharing between two intentional selves, each with mental lives is different as described by Kleinman, myself, and Mattingly. Yet, we all agree that it is the social context and practices that structure these authentic relationships. As I said, we agree more than we disagree. Again, I place the greater importance on the healing relationship, which might be considered synonymous with an authentic relationship. Kleinman and I agree on this definition.

So far, I've challenged Kleinman's assertion that the doctor has to explore the illness narrative to achieve a healing relationship in medical-surgical clinical encounters. I contend that the doctor, together with his assistants and the patient, have to perform the healing ritual, and the natural consequence of doing that is the doctor and the patient achieve trust and intimacy, the antidote to alienation. Kleinman describes the "Patient Explanatory Model":

> This alternative approach originates in the *reconceptualization of medical care* [emphasis added] as (1) empathic witnessing of the existential experience of suffering and (2) practical coping with the major psychosocial crises that constitute the menacing chronicity of that experience. The work of the practitioner includes the sensitive solicitation of the patient's and the family's stories of the illness, the assembling of a mini-ethnography of the changing contexts of chronicity, informed negotiation with alternative lay perspectives on care, and what amounts to a brief medical psychotherapy for multiple, ongoing threats and losses that make chronic illness so profoundly disruptive.
>
> (1988: 10)

I claim that no reconceptualization of medical care is needed: The healing ritual has withstood the test of time and meets the needs of the patient. Now I would like to consider the remaining portions of Kleinman's Patient Explanatory Model. Exploring the illness (Step 1) could be equated with exploring the diagnosis in a different temporal context. Then Kleinman gives the following outline:

Step 2: The second step in the explanatory model technique is the presentation of the practitioner's explanatory model. No doctor is taught how to explain the biomedical account to patients. Yet that is an essential task in the work of doctoring . . .

Step 3: He must encourage the patient and family members to respond to his model . . .

Step 4: The clinician engages in self-reflective interpretation of the interests, biases, and emotions that underlie his own model.

(Kleinman 1988: 240–243)

Step 2 and Step 3 correlate well with diagnosis narrative and joint attention to the diagnostic narrative, both elements of the healing ritual I described. In fact, the similarity to the healing ritual is striking.

Summary

In contrast to Kleinman's broad approach, I studied the very narrow confines of the Western biomedical clinical encounter in a urology practice. I was looking for "the narrator," and how the story was constructed. That is where I discovered an overlooked "narrative," the diagnosis narrative. The healing ritual involves the construction of the diagnosis narrative as well as "persuasion" of the patient that the diagnosis is correct. This persuasion is not a form of aggression, as so commonly presented, because the biomedical model is a shared cultural practice by both patient and doctor. "Persuasion" as used within the ritual of a current existential threat by helping the patients recognize something about themselves that they already agree with – biomedical science. Persuasion as used by Kleinman allows the doctor to help patients realize something about themselves within the symbolic cultural domain that healer and patient share. Based on my theoretical review, I am describing the narrative structure of shared experience during a healing ritual, expanding on Mattingly's observations of narrative structure of experience. This shared experience is a form of "the ratchet effect" described by Tomasello. I further argue that shared experience creates healing relationships. I argue that healing is a product of the relationship created by the shared experience of the healing ritual. We all agree, however, that more healing in medical practice is a desired goal. I propose an integrative perspective where Mattingly, Kleinman, and I all describe how those healing relationships arise from ritual healing, distinguished by the temporal location of the existential threat. W.H.R. Rivers described a time when religion, medicine, and jurisprudence were undifferentiated in society. In this world of the past, healing would have been called the sacrament of belonging – the antidote for alienation.

Note

1 National Conference for Physician-Scholars in the Social Sciences and Humanities, Harvard Medical School, Boston, April 29–30, 2017.

References

Arendt, Hannah. 1958. *The Human Condition*. Chicago: University of Chicago Press.

Bourdieu, Pierre, and Jean-Claude Passeron. 1990 [1970]. *Reproduction in Education, Society and Culture*. R. Nice, transl. London: Thousand Oaks.

Kleinman, Arthur. 1980. *Patients and Healers in the Context of Culture: An Exploration of the Borderland Between Anthropology, Medicine, and Psychiatry*. Berkeley: University of California Press.

———. 1988. *The Illness Narratives – Suffering, Healing, and the Human Condition*. New York: Basic Books.

———. 2014. The Art of Medicine: How We Endure. *Lancet* 383:119–121.

Leach, Edmund. 1976. *Culture and Communication: The Logic by Which Symbols Are Connected*. Cambridge: Cambridge University Press.

Mattingly, Cheryl. 1998. *Healing Dramas and Clinical Plots: The Narrative Structure of Experience*. Cambridge: Cambridge University Press.

Tambiah, Stanley. 1977. The Cosmological and Performative Significance of a Thai Cult of Healing through Mediation. *Culture, Medicine, and Psychiatry* 1:97–132.

Turner, Edith. 1992. *Experiencing Ritual: A New Interpretation of African Healing*. Philadelphia: University of Pennsylvania Press.

18 Reflections of a healer

In a different genre of scientific writing, this section is the *discussion*. It is the part of a research report where the author says what he or she thinks the significance and meaning of the data, results, and analysis are and how that contributes to our understanding of the world. In the methods section, I mentioned that I would specify when I was speaking as an anthropologist and when I was speaking as a doctor. From the perspective of an anthropologist, the answer to the research question was unexpected. This project also helped me become a better doctor.

When I was collecting data and doing analysis, I disciplined myself to operate strictly as an anthropologist. I find it ethically troubling when physician anthropologists use their own patients in scholarly work. As a physician, your primary obligation is to the patient – the conflict of interest is too great to do otherwise. Research requires informed consent. Physician anthropologists cannot obtain informed consent after the fact. For that reason, I'm informing my readers that this section is different than those before – it's the discussion section and I'm reflecting on the research project, using my data and my experiences with my own patients to convey what I think the meaning of my findings actually are.

I am a medical anthropologist. I am also an anthropological physician. Physicists will tell you that matter is simultaneously both a particle and a waveform. Likewise, I am simultaneously both a medical anthropologist and anthropological doctor. For the purposes of validity, I intellectually separated those domains. For the purpose of discussion, I will be both simultaneously.

In the previous chapter, I reviewed the work of Arthur Kleinman and Cheryl Mattingly and tried to point out the common theoretical foundations. In this section, I hope to explain how each of the three of us described the same social practice from three separate perspectives. I will use the trope of "a story has a beginning, middle, and end."

I believe Kleinman, Mattingly, and I all described healing rituals. The difference is that the existential threat occurred in the past, present, or future. Biomedicine is appropriate only for those existential threats in the present. It is the inability of most doctors to recognize that a healing ritual intended for the present is inappropriate for an existential threat in the past or future that has drawn such criticism from medical anthropologists. This is a valid criticism, which I believe should spark a paradigm shift in medical education. At the same time, I have little regard for doctors who cannot make an accurate biomedical diagnosis.

The experience of doing this research changed me as an anthropologist and as a doctor. I wrote the initial draft of the theory section several years ago. At that time, I intellectually reported that a story can be latent and pre-exist prior to the experience and that experiences from one's past are told as stories. The intellectual integration of the work of Kleinman, Mattingly, and my data arose more recently in my efforts to answer the research question. Using my theoretical frame, my understanding of healing was latent, but now I can tell this story as a reflection – a contemplated past. I could not recognize my actions as a doctor until I viewed them from the perspective of an anthropologist. I confess that for years some of Kleinman's statements infuriated me; now I treasure the nugget of gold in his work that I am able to see in my own work as a doctor. That would have never happened if I had not done this ethnographic work.

The Kleinman procedure

I see outpatients and inpatients at teaching institutions. The medical students and residents occasionally get frustrated and judgmental when a patient refuses to follow the expected biomedical "ritual." When I walk into the patient's room, I listen and assess the temporality of the existential threat. In the hallway, I ask them, "What's the diagnosis?" Invariably, they all offer an implausible biomedical diagnosis – so implausible, the patient cannot recognize it as relevant to their own experience. When the diagnosis is wrong, the healing ritual is a failure. I tell the residents and medical students that the *real* diagnosis is "a distressed soul." The existential threat occurred in the past or imagined future – only the suffering is in the present of these clinical encounters. Instead of ordering more CT scans and prescribing more medications, I demand "twenty minutes of unstructured listening." My rules state, "the doctor is not allowed to speak." "Listening" is the appropriate diagnostic test for suffering related to an unresolved existential threat in a patient's past or future. The team usually assigns this task to a medical student with the expectation that the group needs a report on morning rounds the next day. The next day, I always follow up and ask, "What did the patient say?" Uniformly when I have diagnosed a distressed soul, the medical student returns with an illness narrative of epic proportions. Alternatively, they report a story of an intolerable anticipated future. I can see and feel the change in attitude and increased empathy within the rounding group. Compassionate care ensues. Conflict diminishes.

In my clinical practice, the diagnosis of a "distressed soul" occurs less than 5 percent of the time. To elicit illness narratives when someone is facing a life and death situation in the present is inappropriate. It is equally inappropriate to continue to push the biomedical healing ritual when the diagnosis is incorrect.

Many surgeons who develop a new surgical procedure attach their name to the procedure. I gave an example of this in Chapter 11. Surgeons need to know when to do the procedure and when it is contraindicated. This decision is often determined by an anatomical diagnosis. I wish medical schools would teach students when it is appropriate to do a "Kleinman procedure" for a patient. Michael Balint wrote how to make that diagnosis, and John Salinsky described the procedure in his book *The Last Appointment: Psychotherapy in General Practice* (1993).

For other difficult patients, I diagnose "social death." These patients have circumstances where there are no social connections that make life worth living. It carries a horrible prognosis. These patients need a "Mattingly procedure." Medical learners are often skeptical, but I can easily distinguish these different patient presentations. Again, I lament that medical education limits skill acquisition; patient care would be greatly enhanced if the work of Mattingly and Kleinman was understood and applied appropriately.

Recall in Chapter 13 the patient who kept insisting, "I know my body." During that office visit, Dr. Jeffries kept suggesting biomedical diagnoses and the patient kept rejecting them. The doctor and the patient shared a negative attachment to each other. I remember my feet hurt because the office visit was so long. Had that patient showed up in my office, I would have diagnosed a distressed soul and done a Kleinman procedure. I would have made sure I was sitting before embarking on that venture. Remember though, this case was the one exception to hundreds of office visits where the biomedical healing ritual was efficacious. Yet, anthropologists learn from the exceptions to the rules as well as usual practice.

Biomedical healing rituals

I teach evidence-based medicine and clinical epidemiology at the medical school. I am amazed at how often doctors get the diagnosis wrong. Based on my research, this is not only expensive, but is associated with a terrible human toll for patients. Recall Susan Greenhalgh's experience. The *Wall Street Journal* put a dollar price tag on incorrect diagnoses; there is a cost to society.

When I said I became a better doctor, I became more aware of how much patients need a specific diagnosis. For many years, I would teach the residents and medical students that when they saw a patient with headaches, they must tell the patient that they do not have a brain tumor. I learned this by trial and error, but it is a good example that gives face validity to my research. It did not help the patient much to tell them they had a tension headache. It was also necessary to tell them they did not have a brain tumor – this was always the unexpressed existential threat initiating the office visit. When I tell patients this, there is usually a sigh of relief and lightening of the mood. I suppose people can deal with a headache, but when they are scared (for whatever reason) that it might be something more, they go to the doctor. Repeatedly, patients reveal how scared they were and what a relief it was to know their health was not at risk only after they know they don't have a brain tumor.

In primary care, we try to use the diagnostic label "viral chest cold" so patients do not seek inappropriate antibiotics. After this research, I add, "That means that you do not have pneumonia." I typically give the patient both the medical version of a diagnosis and a layman's translation with the significance for them. I also "diagnose" chronic conditions with a status assessment of their diabetes or heart problem. Dr. Spangler did this almost routinely because she was managing prostate cancer as a chronic disease. I do this now because I recognize that the diagnosis helps the patient understand why the treatment suggested is important. It is an American habit to want to "fix things" when in fact, most patients probably need the diagnosis before they change behavior.

Doing a "Mattingly procedure" in clinical practice

I have already spoken about how much I admire Cheryl Mattingly for her theoretical advancement in anthropology. Her work also has the potential to have a major impact on clinical practice of medicine. I find Mattingly's description to be quite similar to motivational interviewing. The interaction focuses on finding a culturally acceptable way to live life given severe limitations.

Each time a doctor and patient go through a healing ritual together, the doctor-patient relationship strengthens. Eventually it becomes a healing relationship. I cared for a woman who had many hospitalizations for heart failure. One day in the office, I said to her, "You know everyone has to die sometime. Tell me about what you want that day to be like for you." We sat and talked for a long time. I allowed this patient to "locate desire" for her imagined future life. Nine months later, I saw her again in the hospital and she told me, "Do you remember that conversation we had in the office a while back? That day has arrived." I told her to call her daughters so they could participate while the patient withdrew care. The next day on rounds, I could tell there was tension in the air. Her daughters were upset. Apparently, the patient and her family had not shared with each other what the patient had shared with me. While speaking to the patient, I said, "You remember our conversation." I simply repeated the conversation with the patient again in the presence of her daughters. I then said, "So what you told me was you no longer want to pursue active treatment and you think now is the time for hospice." The patient confirmed that aloud. I was already down the hall seeing other patients and one of the daughters ran up to me, crying, and said, "Thank you so much. I could never have lived with myself had

I not heard Mom say it herself." A few months later, I got a note letting me know the patient had died and thanking me for making her last few months such a wonderful family time. All I did was a "Mattingly procedure" that day in the office.

Again, when I was presenting data, recall the man who saw Dr. Stein for follow-up. He had been to three health systems and Dr. Stein told him what others had already told him. That man needed to grieve the loss of his functional body. His erectile dysfunction, inability to empty his bladder, and incontinence are the equivalent of a spinal cord injury. He needed an empathic witnessing of *sadness, fear, guilt*, and *anger* (I label them the "fab four"). I find these four emotions are semantic clusters of emotional cognitions. After grieving (Kleinman procedure), the doctor should do a "Mattingly procedure" for that particular patient. "You said yourself that you a young man. That means you have a lot of life yet to live. None of us have the life we wanted, but we all have to find our way. What do you imagine doing a year from now, five years from now, or before you die?"

The work of a healer

In the methods section I typed out the words, "I am a master clinician," and I thought that sounded like a braggart, so I deleted them. Staring at the blank page, I eventually retyped those same words.

In the previous section, I told a story about a patient with congestive heart failure. I used it as an example from my clinical practice of healing as described by Cheryl Mattingly. Additionally, I formulated the diagnosis and performed healing rituals for an existential threat in the present many times. "Your congestive heart failure is worse on today's exam. I know you'll be disappointed, but I recommend you go back to the hospital for a few days." After multiple episodes of healing rituals of that type, a healing relationship develops, which is the only reason I was able to so easily diagnose impending end of life, initiating a "Mattingly procedure" of locating desire of an imagined future with limited options. Also within the context of that relationship, it is normal for a person to review the life they have led. I performed multiple Kleinman procedures with that patient as well. "Tell me about when you were a child." "So how did you handle that challenge?" "How do you think that affected your life?" "Do you think that affects your life today?" "What do you think has been left unsaid that your daughters need to know?"

I have argued that "healing" as described by Arthur Kleinman, Cheryl Mattingly, and me are three versions of healing rituals with slightly different forms based on the location in time of the existential threat. A true healer seamlessly weaves back and forth, even within the same clinical encounter. That is what I do.

Unfortunately, medical education often emphasizes only a biomedical model. In fairness, it requires a lot of specialized knowledge to make accurate diagnoses. Doctors should not have to learn how to be healers through a lifetime of experience; they should receive mentoring early in their careers. A coherent, comprehensive anthropological explanation of healing would have tremendous pragmatic value to doctors and patients.

What is healing?

The research question was "What is healing?" When I began my research, the dominant anthropological answer was narrating a life story into a coherent "self." I discovered a completely different answer – it has nothing to do with constructing a self, something I tried to show is latent and exists primordially at birth. Rather, healing is about the relationship between self and society. To define healing, I looked at the "story arc" of the ritual story. This story starts with a person facing the existential threat of disease and death, a form of impending annihilation. Whatever relationship to society that person had changes immediately. Following the ritual taxonomy, the person is forced into the realm of "anti-structure," a form of alienation from their former life, but also from a full functional member of society. Thus, anti-structure is a threat to both the self and society. Scary and painful things happen during this time of anti-structure, often imposed by the "tribal elders." Yet, the goal is not to harm, but to transform. The doctor acts as guide and mentor for learning a new way of life that can be reintegrated into our culture as a person with a new social position. This rite of passage is called life. Therefore, the one sentence answer to my research question is:

> *Healing is the ritual process where a "self" facing annihilation by an existential threat of disease navigates the liminal social space of alienation from the cultural body and reconnects with a new cultural role by forming a healing relationship with the socially authorized healer – the doctor.*

Appendices

Appendix A
Individual patient narratives

This section records the personal narratives of three patients. I obtained the data with ethnographic interviews. Because the patients were speaking to the researcher privately (not in a clinical care setting), the context changes the content and style. In many ways, this methodological change highlights how illness narratives exist outside the cultural practices of a clinical office visit. I expect language use to be different in an office setting compared to a private retelling – context matters because there are different cultural rules of communication between the two settings. These interviews were digitally recorded monologues – each respondent talked reflectively and extensively without prompts. These verbalizations lack the structure of a conversation or the structure of an interview. I decided to transcribe their verbalizations as close to "natural speech" as possible, so there will be small gaps, redundancies, jumps, and logical lapses. The intent is to have the "individual voice" be heard without filters. In this way, these data are complementary to the participant observation.

The patient interviews are a form of illness narratives – they include topics not found in the clinical encounter or the social spaces of the clinical encounter. Thus, they describe the patients' lived experiences. Note however, the patients have incorporated aspects of the healing ritual into their stories.

Paul's story

To me the beginning was the results of a physical exam that had a PSA test that was slightly elevated above normal. I don't remember whose idea it was to draw the PSA. I don't think I ever requested it. Although I do remember having a discussion. Well I don't – It showed up. So I think it was something that the doctor – Gossett Family Physicians is where we go. He said now that I was 50, that this was something we should start screening for.

So I was now 51 and so it was something that should be, we should be screening for. And I remember being a little perturbed because I went back the year before and just looked up my blood tests and it wasn't run. So it occurred because I'd hit a magical age of 50 and I was a little taken aback,

I guess because I'm thinking well I hit 50, and they did the first test and it was positive, so shouldn't we have been screening at some time before now to be sure we caught it and as it turned out it was just in time?

It wasn't real high but it was above something that warranted follow-up so . . . and this was with my local doctor. It was a little concerning. It happened right before Christmas one year, whatever year that was. I think I got a letter in the mail – it was just the report with the PSA that they send out the results of the blood test and everything and it was, that was flagged and the comments of "please call me" or something and "we'll follow up on it." That, that was the first little "Okay there's something going on here." At that point it was just the PSA is a little high so I wasn't too wigged out about that, and again I didn't have the benchmark necessarily to compare it to, so I didn't know if it was on a long slow track or on a spike so, I tried not to get too concerned about that. Well, after we talked, he referred me to a specialist.

I think I met with him once and then we came back for the exploratory biopsy, which was interesting. It was all very innocuous and how it was approached. "We're just going to insert this little thing in here, just kind of look around and if I see something I don't really like then I may just take a little nip of it." Well, it was the first little nip of it that was truly a nip of my prostate, which was slightly painful.

Well, you're always thinking – well I'm, you're back and forth. It's not gonna be me. Or yeah well maybe it is. And then my entire life is gonna change. So you're back and forth, I was back and forth between, okay I'm gonna deny that this is happening or I'm gonna accept it and get all wigged out and that's going to be too difficult to handle so I'm gonna go back here and say you know statistically I'm sure this is not me. And so we just move on. And I don't remember how long it was, I don't recall it as being an extended period of time, it was within a few days I think . . .

I think he, it was a follow-up office visit, that once I'd gone in and then he had done the biopsy and then when I came back I think I got a phone call to come in and sit down and go through the results. And that came back positive. I think it was four of seven samples were positive for cancer and it was deemed to be a fairly aggressive form of it at the time. From all they could tell it was contained within the prostate. I had a discussion with the surgeon afterwards . . . okay, how long do I have before it got beyond the prostate because it was all contained within the prostate which was one of the things I attribute to a good outcome and everything. "Ok, well, how long did I have?" "Certainly six months. Maybe a year." But it was a fairly aggressive growing form of cancer. But his characterization of it was, it's a Gleason 7 . . . I think it was seven, and that was on the higher end of the aggressive scale, it wasn't the most aggressive. But it was getting towards that point which meant it was – what it meant to me was it was a fairly fast-growing thing that isn't something you would sit there and do nothing with because it's, something else is gonna kill you first. It was something that should be treated was the message I was getting because of my age that I had a great life span left and the cancer was fairly aggressive and so the two were not compatible. So something needed to be done about it.

When the specialist said yeah you do have cancer. You go, "Hm." That was kind of a wake-up call. I was pretty young and certainly, and I had no symptoms. None. Nothing, no blood, no large prostate. No problems going to the toilet. No nothing. So it was pretty much out of the blue that there was even anything recognized, that there was anything wrong. So that was a little bit of a setback or at least a concern.

Well, I knew enough about what was going on to know that prostate surgery included urinary incontinence and sexual problems and things and so you're imagining, I'm gonna run around with a diaper for the rest of my life and my sex life is just gone completely and is gonna stop from here on and I'm gonna to be rendered pretty much unable to do any of that. I mean, that's, you jump to the extreme of what you've heard and know about.

So I think I met again with them to, a doctor to go over treatment options and that type of thing and the basic consensus was for someone of my age, which was 50 at the time – 51 – that I should think about surgery as the option rather than radiation or some other passive wait-and-see type of treatment. I don't remember his exact words, but it was laid out in, within the context of I'm a relatively young man, I'm 51, at my age he would recommend the surgery as the best form of treatment because I have a long life yet to live and some of these other things are not, don't get rid of it and could lead to more things down the road if radiation doesn't quite do it or there's some complications with radiation. And there was also certainly complications with, potential complications with the surgery, but it was the goal of getting rid of it. Fixing it. Getting rid of it. The cancer. And the way to get rid of it was surgery. Everything else it's still there and it's, we're treating it, and we're managing it, but it's still there. For somebody your age, I'd lean towards getting rid of it.

A colleague of my wife had a husband that had been through similar things more advanced and more serious than what I was dealing with and he had a very positive experience at the University and referred me there. My thinking at the time and the reason for going to Dr. Monty was he had at least I had become aware and some of it was from the reference that got me there. And other sources, I don't recall. He had developed some surgical techniques that went out of their way to not just hack away at it and take whatever was left. His specialty was leaving as many of the nerves as possible and being very exact in how this was done and he has developed a reputation for that and with some very good results. His whole focus was we're gonna do this and leave you in absolutely the best shape we can to live a normal life from here on. And so that aspect of it, of the outcomes was pretty high in my looking for, you know, I wanted it to be a successful surgery but my mission was I want it to be successful. And I want my full function of my body when I'm all done and so the whole emphasis on, the whole reason for going to Dr. Monty was the, . . . I'll say reputation, but it was the focus of a lot of his research and his practice was doing this surgery in as least harmful way as possible.

I don't remember at what point we heard from this friend of ours and it was probably at the point we knew we had it, but before we had decided where we were gonna do and how we were gonna go about this. So I know there were some questions about, okay how many of these do you do? And it was something like well 20 or 25 a year. And then we were comparing that with Dr. Monty, who did 30 a week or something like that, it was drastically different the number of these things that people did. And so that was also part of the discussion of where we were gonna have this done and how we were gonna do it.

So I contacted Dr. Monty over there who was the surgeon who had done the other guy's surgery and for seeking at least a second opinion and potentially to do the surgery. Well, he was very busy and it was going to be very difficult to get in to see him. I think he was the head of the oncology department over there and so getting to Dr. Monty was supposed to be rather difficult and the first contact was, "well, you know, would you be interested in having one of his students or one of his colleagues do that?" And I said, "I really would like to have Dr. Monty do this" and subsequently I was accepted as a patient of Dr. Monty and met with him at least once to go over that and then ultimately the surgery was scheduled.

I had told the head of the company, local head of the company, and the people in the office all knew. My boss in Detroit came to visit me just as I was leaving the next day. And I told, the people at church knew. It was, it was very difficult to tell people I have cancer. It was probably the most difficult, leading up to the surgery that was the most difficult thing about it was telling other people that I had cancer and that I was gonna have to beat this. And it was harder amongst friends than it was at work. Work I had to because I was gonna be gone and I had to plan for that. And I knew when it was gonna be. And so I had an obligation to let them know and we had to plan for it at work. Friends it was just I gotta tell you this, so . . .

It was probably I guess now in thinking about it was one of the most traumatic parts about the whole thing was to tell people I had cancer and that I was gonna have surgery. We would go, kinda made the rounds to our good friends and you know, I think well somehow in the course of conversation we'll, we'll work it into the conversation. Well, it isn't something that comes up in conversation. So we would go over to somebody's house and we'd be there all night and we hadn't said it and I hadn't said anything and I was kinda, [Meg – his wife] was trying to help me a little bit and I was kinda waiting for her to well, Paul's got something to tell ya. Or something to say well, by the way, I have prostate cancer. And I was viewing that as a, that was a really difficult thing to tell people that I had cancer and I don't quite know why. It was a flaw in me or something. I don't know. It was, I didn't want to burden them with my problems. I'm not sure I ever really understood that. I mean, I remember we had, I had told Pastor. We had gone to sit down with him and let him know and then the Sunday before the surgery I was on the prayer chain, er . . . on the prayer list. That I was gonna be having surgery and I remember you know I had to run up and tell the guys in the choir, "Well I'm gonna be on the prayer list because I have cancer and I have surgery on Monday." And I had put it off that much and so I was, something I felt I needed tell people, but it was really hard to say, "I've got cancer."

The surgery went well. The second interesting time of the whole experience, first one being the biopsies, was the peeling off of the surgical gauze or adhesive tape that was taped over the incision. The day I was to be discharged, which was I think the next day after the surgery. I might have been there one whole day. It was on a Monday. It might've been Tuesday afternoon and I was leaving. Maybe it was Wednesday. I don't remember. It was no longer than that. Anyhow, one of his residents or support staff came in and said, "Well, everything's looking good, you're ready to go. You can go on home. I just need to take this little bandage off." So he starts peeling this thing off and he's coming at it from both sides and he's saying, "Oh, I'm sorry. Oh, I'm so sorry." And I'm thinking somewhere in modern medicine there has to be a better way to do that but he got the tape off. It was very painful in a very tender area right after surgery. And the guy was so apologetic about the, the guy that came in, and he said well you just have to take this over and he'd pull a little bit from the side and he's oh, I'm sorry. And then he pulled a little bit from this side. Oh, I'm sorry. And then pull a little bit more from the side. And I'm thinking there has to be a better way to do that than to have a completely open wounds from here to there and then to lay this thing across there. Even if you put a little gauze in there between it. But I think it was solid gauze all the way or solid adhesive all the way across. And I think he actually did and I still have just a little bit of a scar tissue where one of the staples or something kinda pulled out a little bit when he pulled this thing out. And so it just struck me as there, with all the sophistication of everything had been the way to bandage the thing up was to just to lay this thing across the open wound and then rip it off a day later.

Then I laid there for a little while and recovered from that experience and then we came on home. I was out of work three weeks. I was in the hospital a couple of days. I think I went back to work part time I think the third week after. And there were a couple of days there that okay it's noon and I'm going home. So I think I was off two weeks, and then the next week I was kind of part-time and then after that I was back to work pretty normally. I mean the first five or six days I have the catheter and so I want to get that out and that was a step. And there was oh I don't know, it was probably a couple of months I was still wearing diapers to just make sure I was gradually gain urinary control again and so I would say six months I was pretty much over the whole thing.

But Dr. Monty's observation of the prostate afterwards that they felt that the outer wall of it had not been penetrated by any cancer cells and then that was confirmed, at least the, what was portrayed to me as confirmation was that two weeks later my PSA was now less than 0.1 or less than whatever the detection limit was and it has remained there since. I get a PSA once a year now just as part of my regular physical. Dr. Monty's, I followed up with him for about five years and basically said there's no reason to continue to follow up so when I get my blood tests with my regular physical we still send a copy to Dr. Monty but there's no further follow-up with him.

Well, most of the time I don't think about it much. A lot of the time I, I felt like I came through it really, really well to the point where I live my life virtually completely normally since and I've had the thought that I really you know that people will talk about being cancer survivors and I, my image of cancer survivors are people who have been through hell and back and still have pain or have some pretty devastating things that they are dealing with on a regular basis and I don't have any of that. And so I don't feel like a cancer survivor. I'm not a real one at least. Mine was, yeah it was a scare. And it wasn't particularly pleasant to have it, the surgery and everything. I wouldn't choose to go through it again but once I was done with it, I was pretty well done with it and have continued to, like I say I lead a quite normal life.

The outcome overall has been very good. My PSA has been less than 0.1 for over 10 years now. I have very few if any side effects as a result of it. Overall, I've certainly been very pleased with the outcome that has resulted from it. I recommended him to at least one other good friend of mine who has done the same route with Dr. Monty based on my recommendation.

It's much easier now because it's all behind me and it's all worked out really well. I can look back on it, again I think you – it was an unknown, it was the fear of the unknown, I don't know what's gonna happen, I don't know how this is gonna turn out. After the fact when it's turned out really well, it's much easier to relate, and say, "You know, I had a very positive experience with this after the fact." There were a couple of highlights in there but it was – and you know I, there've been several people that have welcomed me to the club of guys who have had prostate cancer and there were several at church that, "Well, welcome to the club." And I got a little teddy bear or something from one of our friends and, and Pastor, now there was a teddy bear and then there was another little stuffed toy that was a good luck thing, so I've passed it on and it's actually been passed on several times now. I passed it on to Tom, who also had his surgery with Dr. Monty, and then another friend of his, and so he passed it on, and I don't know where it is now. But it was just something that we can kinda did, "Well, okay, I've got a friend who's gonna go through this" and so I'm gonna give him the, it was just a good luck thing, so it was, that was kinda fun.

Tony's story

I have a great internist. And . . . I love my family doctor. And we . . . I had an annual physical and had a whole gamut of tests . . . One of them. . . . One of them is what is called the PSA test, and it came in at one. Okay, that's great. And then about 18 months later I had the same, the same tests, and the PSA came in at five. And she was like, "okay, this is unusual." We laughed about it. She said come in and were going to do the PSA test again. And I said so what, are we going to do the best-of-three? [laughing] And she said, yes something like that. So I went in a second time and it went from . . . It was at 6.3 so then she said, okay now this is serious so she gave me a whole bunch of antibiotics "in case you have an infection. Take these for 21 days and get it tested again" and I just did that just before Labor Day and it was 6.4. At that point, she called me and said you know what, I'm just in internist and I did what I could and, I'm not the specialist. It's time for you to start seeing, . . . the professional.

She referred me to Dr. Stein and made the appointment and that's how I arrived there.

Before the appointment, I checked the internet. Oh, you know, you know, thank God for new technology. It was uh, ha, you could be there for hours and you investigate what PSA is and what it means and what the reading is and then you start reading about prostate cancer and this other stuff and you say, "OK. This is this could be serious."

Well, I knew what the PSA test was . . . It's like, it's kind of like something that leads to, whether or not you have prostate cancer. It's a trigger, yeah it's, what you call it, I don't know. It doesn't mean anything, doesn't mean anything but if A equals B, then *possibly* B equals C.

I didn't know what to expect at the appointment today. I made the appointment and the doctor's office called me yesterday to confirm it . . . and both times I said what do I need to bring? . . . Nothing, . . . okay how do I prepare? Do I need to not eat or anything? . . . Nope, none of that. Well okay, now, so to be honest with you, today's appointment was . . . was one of five in my calendar. And to a very large degree that's the way it's been all week I spent Monday and Tuesday, I was in Toronto on business, Uhmm, I did talk to . . . I had a friend in from Tokyo over the weekend. He was in for business so his family was still in Tokyo so I spent a lot of time with him over the weekend. We talked about it, uhmmm because I emailed him about it, we talked about it a little bit but the gravity of it, the gravity of the whole situation it still, even on the weekend it still didn't hit me. It's like I'll go see what this doctor has to say and we'll go from there type thing.

I'll be honest with you, it wasn't until, it wasn't until I left the office and I was already down in the elevator, I was in the lobby of the building where . . . I wouldn't say I had a mini breakdown, but holy shit, that's when the whole gravity of the potential . . . kind, . . . It kind of flooded on me. That's when it hit me. That was the mini breakdown when I finally got down into the lobby, yes . . . up until then, you know I am a. . . . I'm an automotive engineer.

I work on the premise of data. And without data, you know we have a saying in the engineering world, without data you're just another idiot with an opinion. And when I walked in the office today I had no data. So, it's like there's nothing to worry about here there's nothing to, we're here to gather data and I addressed it, I addressed it, like I said it was one meeting on my calendar out of five today and I addressed it the same way I addressed the other four. And it wasn't a, what word am I looking for . . ., it wasn't a release mechanism, a cover up mechanism, you know it wasn't like I was trying to . . . what word am I looking for? . . . I don't know so I'm so scared about this that I'm then treated like an engineering assignment. I wasn't trying to do that. I just did it. You know the way I attack, attack things.

So after today's appointment . . . Where am I now? I am . . . You know, I got a little bit more data but I still don't have the, well okay let's take the next step. When he [Dr. Stein] said you want to take the next step? It's like of course I want to take the next step. You know when he said . . . let's do the biopsy he said, do you want to it? I didn't get it . . . you want me to say no? I didn't get that. Of course I want to take the next step. We'll probe further – we gotta get data, data, data. We gotta do this. . . . If he would've said we have an opening tomorrow I would have said put me in coach. I'm like, let's keep going let's keep going. I'm like, let's keep going.

I'm not, I'm not as much . . . Where I am right now at whatever time it is, nine o'clock I'm not as, I'm past the breakdown stage and I'm into let's keep going, let's figure this thing out. Let's go coach. I have to wait for the biopsy and then I wait for the report, [laughing] 10 days to two weeks after that. And you know it's not like I'm going to be sitting drumming my fingers on the table, it's going be like okay get on with my life, it's not going to be like let's go skydiving now, let's go mountain climbing, no no no when it's in the calendar let's do it.

[The interview continues the day of the follow up visit after the biopsy.]

Well, the results are negative. And at the end of the day that's kind of anti-climactic in that – I'm starting in my car here, [laughs] that's going on. You know, had the biopsy and they told me the results would be ready in a week. And he said what the doctor said, what would you like us to do? You want us to schedule a follow-up appointment? And I said, hell no, I want you to call as soon as those results hit the mailbox. And they did, they called me and I had the biopsy on a Wednesday and they called me on a Monday.

Yeah, actually Dr. Stein called me, yeah. And he left me a voicemail. And it was, you know, "Hello Tony, this is Dr. Stein calling, you said you wanted to know as soon as possible about the results. I'm just calling to let you know the results are negative and the next steps are to keep a watch on this and come back in a year, and we'll see what happens." All on a voice mail.

Okay. [laughs] – I did call the office and ask Marsha to send my results to my internist; she did that.

I saw my internist last week. I got the results on Monday and just serendipity I had an appointment with my internist on Thursday. She was all happy, congratulations, don't have cancer. And she the internist basically said she gave me a little bit more detail, you don't have this or this either, which is good news, and these are kind of precursors of cancer and there was no evidence of that either. So that's good news. And then the internist said basically the same thing, okay we're going to keep our eye on this from now on. And keep our eye on it. . . . it doesn't bother me, it doesn't make me happy, it doesn't make me sad. It is what it is. My cardiologist, when I went to him, he actually said, "Welcome to the new club." I said, "What club is that?" "Medicated for life club." [laughter] It's kind of everything, the cardiologist, the medicated for life, the colonoscopy, the cancer biopsy, the prostate scare, all of this is kind of like yeah, well, you know what, you aren't 21 anymore. You know? It's funny, not funny, but I talk about these things with my buddies, who I've been friends with since high school, and yeah, it's not like their eyes get wide and it's like, "S**t, not you!" They're like, "Oh yeah, I have a colonoscopy too." But gee, the subjects change when you're 50 I guess. [laughs]

I'll be honest with you, when he told me that there was about a – he told me it was about 50/50. When I walked in there to get the biopsy I said, "Okay, doc, I'm sure you haven't thought about this since I walked out of the room two weeks ago but it's the only thing I've thought about. Now that you've seen me, you read the chart, you've had the first little go-around," I said, "What does your gut say?" "50/50." I said, "Oh, great." Because between the initial consultation and the biopsy I did a little bit more research. And that was not pretty. It was like, I don't want this. The two weeks was tough because, like I said, I did some more investigation about well, what if the results come back positive, and it was like I said it was not pleasant. And then of course the week in between, between the biopsy and the results is now you're on needles.

The biopsy . . . It's funny because my internist is a female, and apparently, I don't know, I don't even know if they've got a prostate gland, I don't know. She said, she said to me, interestingly, she had a patient today, one of her patients who did the same thing, and he said, it was the most pain he felt in his life. She's like, "Was it really that bad?" And I'm like, "No, it was not the most pain I've felt in my life. It was not pleasant, but it was not the most pain." And what they do, and the doctor tells you, he puts an anesthesia on the gland itself. Kind of like a dentist when he numbs your tooth, you put the local anesthesia right where he needs it. Okay, but that doesn't help the instrument going up your butt, you know. Which again, you know what, not pleasant but not horrible, right. It's when the anesthesia wears off, because it's up there, you can't, you can't – you know what, you can't do anything, you can't touch it, you can't squeeze it, you can't – oh, so my doctor said, "What did it feel like?" And I had the best answer. I said, I said, "Take a beer bottle, a longneck like a Bud Light." "Yeah, okay." "Leave the cap on." "Okay." "Shove it up your butt and twist it around. That's what it feels like."

Yeah. And it was I'd never done this in my life. You get the procedure done, it's ten minutes, it's not long. And you've got the anesthesia, like a dentist, well the dentist numbs your tooth and works on it for ten minutes, you pop out of that chair saying, okay, see you later. And that's kind of what I did. And then it wore off. I actually drove to a pharmacy, but by this time it's nine o'clock at night. And I said, "I just had a prostate biopsy." And the pharmacist said, "Okay, where's your prescription." It's like, "He didn't give me one." She's like, "Uh-oh."

I remember the beer bottle, I remember it was painful, I remember the relief when I found out it was negative. I'm thrilled I don't have cancer. [laughs] And as much as I researched it and it was ugly and everything else, you know what, you don't want to go through that door. You don't want to think oh shit, I might actually really have cancer – you just can't accept it until you get the news. Again, as much as you research it, everything else, it's like no, this isn't going to happen to me. This is bad and I don't want it to happen to me. It's not going to happen. You almost you could will it away, you try. So then when it comes it's like yes.

Alfred's story

Well, I was – I always have blood tests. I have had colon cancer and they took out a foot of colon. And I went through 14 months of chemotherapy. So I've always had blood tests periodically and in that they included the PSA. The PSAs were low and all of a sudden the numbers started to climb. When they climbed to a certain level my personal physician said I think you should go see a urologist. Which I did and the urologist said well, based on your numbers I would like to take a biopsy. So I said okay let's do that. So they took a biopsy and they found out that there were areas of malignancy in the prostate. So the doctor – Jones was his name – the urologist, well I can take care of it so forth and so forth. I said no, I'd rather go to Belmont. I'm a member of the Belmont Society and my whole family has contributed heavily to, to Belmont over the years. I went there and talk to the people in their oncology department and I felt it was really quite unsatisfactory, or felt unsatisfactory the way I was being treated there and their attitude of the oncologists and surgeons there. One surgeon right away said we're gonna cut it out. I said oh oh no you're not. I want to hear the whole story because they had given me a paper, a document and it said that there were several methods of handling prostate cancer – cryotherapy, radiation, surgery, something to do with herbs and so forth. And I read through it and I said, I want to explore my options.

As it turned out later I found out that the people, the doctors I was talking to at Belmont were planning on leaving Belmont and they did not fulfill their obligation to the patients coming in to Belmont's oncology department at that particular time. I'm sorry I didn't, wasn't able to go to Belmont. Because, as I say, my family is very close to Belmont. You walk in the Green Oak office, main building and our names are on the wall in gold letters because we contributed and you figure well, you certainly would go to the place where you give money to and have a lot of faith in. But it had to be explained to me later through the foundation that these people were leaving and they slipped up. And it rebuilt my confidence in them, but I'm satisfied. I'm not sorry that I went to Connaught and my family will be considering them in, for gifts of financial help in the future.

I think it was nine or ten doctors that left. All left on their own. And the administration of Belmont did send letters and I got mine explaining what happened. That there were other people complained. It could've been handled a little bit better. It's just a – you know that I had to call them for everything. When is my appointment? Well, what am I supposed to do? And they wouldn't return calls. It was just, I had the feeling that they were disorganized. Well I wasn't not about to place my body in the hands of a bunch of disorganized people. And it's unfortunate and explain that to administrators at Belmont and they said oh my God. They explained that these people were leaving; they're setting up their own practice. But you don't treat patients that way. I wouldn't go to them now for any amount of money.

So, based on comments made by people in the condo complex that I [live], and a friend of mine also had been to Connaught for prostate cancer, Well, this one doctor, very nice, well I'm a surgeon and we could cut it out and so forth. And I thought, I said I want to hear more. And thinking a couple of the elderly men here in our complex had it removed and they've had to wear diapers constantly. So when I talked to Dr. Rivers, I liked the way his approach was and I wanted to try something different. I was not about just have it whacked out and then end up wearing a diaper.

I was at Connaught maybe oh I don't know a couple hours for my first appointment. I can't remember the name of the first doctor I met, that was the surgeon, and then they said, well, Dr. Rivers will come in and talk to you also. I spoke to him. Then finally I said, that's the way I would like to go. I want to try radiation.

I went over to see Dr. Rivers at Connaught Cancer Center. In fact, I've met several doctors there and I convinced myself based on previous experience – I've had basal cell carcinoma of the nose, and they did a wonderful job with radiation – I thought I would have radiation done as it was explained to me there at Connaught Cancer Center. And the doctor, the oncologist explained to me what would be the side effects [of what] they thought. I was mostly concerned with ending up with a diaper. I've seen too many men my age and my complex here who are either having to wear a diaper or they're dribbling or one problem after another. And I just was really concerned with that. Dr. Rivers said well what about your sex life. I said at 77 years of age, I don't have a sex life. And that is hardly a thing that is important to me. What is important is the quality of life not having to wear a diaper. So I went through the procedures there; I can't remember whether it was 29 or 32 days of [treatment with] radiation every day. Gosh, they were so professional and so kind and nice and made you feel comfortable when you were in there that it was really easy for me. And I had the entire deal and so far I've had no side effects whatsoever. That's about where I'm at. I feel very comfortable with my life, the way it is. I'm a widower and that part is no problem. My health seems pretty good. That's my story [in a] nutshell.

Well also, I'd had that basal cell carcinoma of the nose and that was an experience in itself. This was done in Florida and I went to this dermatologist. She said well we'll have to cut until we get all the cancer. And I said well, how far you gonna cut? She said I don't know. We'll keep cutting until we know we've got it all. And a lady friend of mine had had the same problem up here in Michigan and she literally ended up a third nostril because they cut and cut and cut and cut. And I said no, I'm going to go to the Moffitt Cancer Center down in Tampa, Florida. This upset the dermatologist quite a bit and I said no, you're just not gonna carve on me. I'm gonna get another opinion. She says well here and she gave me a card and that was this radiation oncologist and he was on a street not too far from where I lived in Tampa Bay. I went to see them and he looked me over and said a few nasty words about the dermatologist. They usually send them to me when they're all carved up. But he said this is one I can handle and it will be a wonder for you. I said what am I gonna look like? He said well for little while you'll look like maybe you drink too much. Your nose is gonna be red. But after that you'll never even know that you had had any problem there. And that was six years ago and you can't even tell that I've had any radiation.

And I was so pleased with it and I thought well, radiation isn't that bad. And you know they've come such a long way in a few years in all kinds of medicine. Back when I moved back to Michigan, I went to see the old oncologist that had given me all this chemotherapy when I had the colon cancer and he looked me over and he said boy you've come a long way and this is super great and everything. And we were talking and he said oh, all that stuff we gave you, we don't do that anymore. That was barbaric. We've come such a long way now. You wouldn't lose your hair, you wouldn't be vomiting all over the place. It would be a totally different world. And they have. In twenty years medicine has come so far, it's unbelievable. And radiation has come a long long way. And I feel very comfortable with it. What told me that was experiences with other people that I've met in my lifetime and their experiences, like when I say this lady friend of mine, they carved her nose up something terrible and even today she looks awful. And I was not about to go that way when the dermatologist said were gonna start carving on your nose. I said oh no you're not. I'm gonna see what other alternatives I have. And when I see, we have breakfast here at Cobblestone

Ridge every other Tuesday and I sit down at this table there sometimes thirty people and a good third of them are elderly men like myself. I would say 80 percent of them have had prostate cancer or problems and the ones who had it removed have all had trouble. They're either dribbling or they're wearing diapers. I thought, wait a minute, I'm not gonna go that way until I find out what the alternative is. And all Dr. Rivers had to say to me is no you will not have to wear a diaper. Well, that convinced me right there.

And I was asking questions like crazy at these breakfasts and they speak up. Yeah no problem at all. One fellow had something called green, what was it, green chemotherapy, I think he called it. And it was a total failure and he still has the cancer and he's going through all kinds of nonsense. Some of them tried diet and different things. Well that's not gonna work. You gotta listen to the professionals and make up your mind which one you're gonna go to. When he said, radiation and no diaper – that was it for me. I felt comfortable with Dr. Rivers. And that he assured me that there would be no after effect. And I don't have any aftereffect. Sure it's some degree of a gamble. You're taking a man's word that really I have no background on him but the people that have been to Connaught gave it the highest praise and my closest friend who had prostate cancer went there and he had radiation only he had the radiation seeds that were permanently implanted.

It certainly was a good experience for me.

Appendix B
Doctors talk about work

The interviews of the doctors occurred about six to nine months after I finished my participant observation. When I listened, I was amazed that they corroborated my observations to the extent that they did. Earlier, I described "triangulation" between the cultural body, the individual body, and the body politic as a measure of validity. These interviews provide that corroboration. Although I don't specifically comment on these narratives to preserve the readers' opportunity to form their own impression of what the participants say, I found evidence for the "existential threat," diagnosis narratives, shared cognitions leading to therapy, healing relationships, as well as aspects of training and competence.

Although medical anthropologists have recorded many patient interviews, these interviews also capture the "lived experience" of doctors. I was amazed, but pleased to find consistency between the doctors' interview data and the data from participant observation.

Again, these interviews were audio recorded and transcribed, resulting in the following monologues. There is no conversational structure. There is no interview structure. I started with a "grand tour" question. After I decided the ethnographic interview reached saturation, I asked one question, which is clearly marked in the transcript.

Dr. Stein's perspective

My work . . . So the beginning part is all about gathering data, and that's the formalized process that we use with history and physical examination, imaging studies, laboratory studies. When you become more experienced you can do that quickly and you can integrate the data in your own mind very quickly. The second part is figuring out the impression and plan or the recommendation or your opinion, which is all kind of the same thing. That boils down to a risk/benefit analysis. You have to communicate the risk/benefit analysis to the patient so that they can make a decision. If the risk/benefit analysis is pretty clear-cut in my mind then I have a more forceful conversation with the patient. If the risk/benefit discussion leaves you in a pretty substantial gray zone, then I'm much less forceful with the patient and consciously try to be less influential.

So let's say the patient's been referred because he was just diagnosed with prostate cancer. So I want to find out what led up to the diagnosis, what did the laboratory study show, what did the biopsy show. Then I want to find out about his urological symptoms and his sexual function symptoms. I want to find out about his general medical history because I need to take into account his overall health in coming to a decision, because prostate cancer occurs in men as they get older and there are a lot of competing factors that come into play. So you have to know about their heart and their lungs. You have to know about their family, you have to know about their sex life. You know, when learning about heart and lungs you want to know is their cholesterol high, do they have diabetes, have they had a heart attack, because that all goes into your mind as to how healthy they are, and that can have a big impact on what you recommend. You get the data by talking to the patient, by looking in the computer, and you often have to struggle to make phone calls, tell your nurse to contact the other hospital, they need to fax something over, it needs to come on a disc, they need to come back next week when we have more information, more data. Sometimes it's easy to gather data, sometimes not. Sometimes the patients are articulate, sometimes they're not. Sometimes they tell you things that you don't need to hear and they go on and on talking about stuff just because they want to talk for whatever psychological reason or need they have, but sometimes what you need you can get pretty quickly and sometimes you can't. But eventually you decide when you have enough data to formulate an opinion.

So for the newly diagnosed prostate cancer patient, one aspect of imaging is do they have metastatic disease? If they do, then you would completely change your treatment plan. For that you rely a lot on what the radiologist said, but you have to look at the images yourself. Radiologists don't really talk to patients, they don't have face-to-face encounters with patients, and they're really kind of technical people that in my opinion they didn't even need to go to medical school to become a radiologist. Of course, people would laugh at me for saying that, and say that I'm completely biased. I understand that. But they basically just sit in a room and look at images, they don't actually even talk to people, for the most part. I'm generalizing and stereotyping, I admit that.

And then the other aspect about imaging for a cancer practice is what's going on with the tumor itself, not the rest of the body. As surgeons, we're very focused on anatomy. We know when an image looks – has certain characteristics, we know what it's going to be like when we go in there and touch it and move it around and cut around it. And again, the radiologists have no idea about that. So what the radiologist says is not very important when you're looking at the surgical aspects of the case. You have to decide – is the surgery going to be easy or hard, is it going to lead to a lot of side effects, are their organs going to be involved? So we really do focus down on the physical characteristics of the tumor itself and the surrounding tissues.

In prostate cancer the patients are all getting older. Maybe some are in their forties, but some are in their fifties, sixties, seventies. Generally the older you get the more likely you are to get prostate cancer. But the older you get the more likely you are to die of something else. So our job is to try to make sure that the patient dies of a heart attack. Or diabetes, or a stroke. So if they have an indolent prostate cancer and they're kind of older, then you can be pretty confident that they're going to die of a heart attack or diabetes or stroke. And that patient you would come to a risk/benefit decision that you're not going to be aggressive about telling them what to do about their prostate cancer, you would tell them don't be so aggressive. A younger patient who has a prostate cancer that has the molecular and cellular characteristics of being aggressive, who has fewer medical problems, like heart disease or diabetes, then you are coming to a decision in your own mind before you even talk to the patient that this patient is far more likely to die and suffer from prostate cancer than the previous patient. When you come to that conclusion in your own mind the conversation you have with that patient is completely different. And you would say things like, "I really think that you should do this or you should do that." Whereas in the first patient you would say, "Well, you can hold off, it's probably – we could do this or we could do that, but I think you don't need to be worried about it, in fact I'd put it out of your mind."

For example, in patients with prostate cancer that you're considering doing a radical prostatectomy, the perfect treatment we call the trifecta, they are cured of cancer, they are potent, and they're continent. And sometimes you can't get a trifecta if they have a large tumor, because in order to get the trifecta you have to preserve nerves and blood vessels that are plastered on to the sides of the prostate. You have to take the prostate out and completely leave those nerves alone, which requires delicate surgery. If they have a big tumor then it's very important to cut the whole tumor out and you want to cut around the tumor, not through it. If you cut through it you'll leave cancer cells behind, which a few years later will turn into a new tumor. So you can get imaging studies of the prostate like an MRI in patients that have bulky, large tumors, try to use the MRI to decide if the sides of the prostate gland are smooth or if they're bulging. And if they're smooth then you can do a better nerve-sparing operation. If it's bulging you might be convinced, you might convince yourself to do a wider operation knowing that you're going to sacrifice some quality of life in order to get the cancer out.

If the computer is nearby and the image is readily available and the patient doesn't have to walk very far, and I think the patient will understand it, then I'll use the images to help the patient understand what I'm going to do and understand the goals and understand why certain aspects of quality of life might be sacrificed. And I often do the same thing with drawings on white pieces of paper in the examination room, to make the same point with a simplified drawing as opposed to a CAT scan.

Active surveillance is a more well-accepted treatment strategy, and I accept it and I promote it. And when patients are diagnosed with certain types of prostate cancer, I often find that I'm the only one in the room telling the patient and his wife and family to calm down, you don't need to do anything fast. Don't let other doctors convince you to have surgery. Just you can safely delay for a number of years and in the meantime enjoy your sex life. So I'm completely in favor of active surveillance in the appropriate patient where in my judgment the patient would not lose any survival by delaying treatment for a number of years.

When I'm having a counseling session with the patient, I'm often the only person in the room – not comparing myself to other doctors but comparing myself to the patient, his wife, sister, brother, family, friends, they're all telling the patient have surgery tomorrow.

So with my professional colleagues there's a spectrum of acceptance of active surveillance. If you give the same scenario to several different people, some people will more strongly go for active surveillance than others, even within my own department. There's different philosophies and different sort of dividing lines about when you would promote active surveillance. And probably if you listen to the conversations between the doctor and the patient behind the closed door of the clinic room you could definitely pick up by the words that we use, that our hand gestures and our eye contact, whether or not we believe what we're saying and how strongly we promote one thing or the other.

How did you get to this place in your career?

I decided to go to medical school because I was good in science and math. I didn't know what else to do, and all my friends in college were going to med school, so I said what the hell, I'll go to med school also. Unlike many other people I had no idea what kind of doctor I wanted to be. When I got into third year med student and started doing all my rotations I liked every single one of them. After a while I decided I liked surgery, I liked the kidney and I liked pelvic surgery, so I decided to go into urology. I don't have father, uncle, brother, anybody else influencing me, I just picked it. Because number one I like surgery, number two I seemed to like what they were doing, but I would have been perfectly happy doing any other kind of surgery, and I probably would have been happy being any other kind of doctor also, except for a radiologist.

I trained in the era before robotic surgery and became a very good open surgeon. And then robotic surgery came along and I thought it would probably be very valuable, so I made a conscious effort to learn how to do it. It took a while to become good at it. I was at the age where I was still able to pick up new things. Hopefully I'm still at that age, fifty-four. Had I been sixty-five or seventy years old maybe I wouldn't have been able to do it. Conversely, younger doctors coming in they're learning robotic surgery and they're not good at open surgery. But I was kind of just at the right time where I was able to overlap both periods so I can do both.

Well, when a big part of your practice is cancer you generally for the most part continue to see the patients for a long time. As opposed to you doing benign surgery where you would see the patient a few times after surgery and then say you don't need to come back anymore. But if someone has cancer there's always a chance that the cancer may come back, so those patients tend to stay in your practice, for the most part. So you often get to know them better than you did before surgery because now you're seeing them at intervals. And when you have a busy surgical practice, before you operate on somebody it's kind of hard to keep them all straight. You get to the operating room at seven o'clock in the morning you have to refamiliarize yourself with the patient, because you're doing it every day. But then when you start to see them in the post-op period and they come back every six months or every three months or something like that, then you start to get to know the patient better. A lot of times I have a closer relationship post-op than pre-op, mainly because you know the patient longer and they tell you about all their personal things, and you try to help them out.

Dr. Jeffries's perspective

When I have a new patient with prostate cancer, they're coming to me with data that must be reviewed prior to me going in there so that I have kind of a mindset and – I don't want to use the word "template," but certainly a counseling framework that I'm going to use when I sit in front of that person and discuss their disease process and what's available to them. So I guess the first step would be to review their materials and kind of risk stratify where their paper data, their objective paper data, places them in the whole stratosphere of prostate cancer, and then start formulating kind of options for therapy. And then I bring those notions or that framework into my interaction with them in the clinical environment, when I engage them.

Oh, so yeah, so my first – if they're an outside referral in I will get a feel for what has been discussed with them, if they fully grasp the reason why they were either referred to me, or if they could explain to me why they sought an opinion from me. Maybe they heard something that they didn't like from their previous physician and they wanted to get another set of eyes on it, or maybe they just are there because their doctor told them that they had to come and see me, and that which is often the case. So once I've established that they know where they are and they have the proper clinical orientation as to the clinical compass as to why they're there and what is the goal of the visit, then I proceed with the goal of the visit, which is an interview, an examination, and usually a very robust discussion about treatment options.

And I don't know what my other colleagues do, but I certainly I value the patient's goals and expectations of treatment very, very highly in terms of the things that we talk about and where we go in terms of treatment.

I think for me to be an effective advocate, I need to have – advocate for the patient – I need to know as much about that patient as I can before I sit in that room and have a conversation with the patient. So if they supply me with data – I think it's a disservice to the patient to walk into the room and go I am so and so, and I'm going to talk to you a little bit about prostate cancer, and do you remember what your PSA is, and this and that. I mean you can do that but I should know those things when I go in there so that I can, you know, really get involved with their care right from the get-go. So yeah, data review, images, laboratories, biopsy results or pathologies, all key to that.

I'm attempting to categorize the patient and their disease into a framework that allows me to sort out people who have potentially lethal disease, or disease that carries with it significant health consequences, from those that have a perhaps non-lethal or subclinical variant of disease. And obviously offer the more aggressive, or counsel the patients to pursue more aggressive curative strategies for those patients that fall into the significant health consequences potentially lethal categories. So when I risk stratify I have that in my mind. A person with a 1 cm equivocal renal mass probably doesn't need their kidney out. But yet their referral and the reason for seeing me is to counsel them as to what do I do with the renal mass, do you know what I mean? So I need to know the imaging data, I need to start working on a clinical gestalt so that I can, again, be an effective advocate for them, and make sure that they are being directed in an appropriate clinical direction.

I can only imagine that they've had a discussion with their primary care doctor, who said Mr. or Mrs. So-and-So, I have some bad news. We got a CAT scan and it reports that you have a mass in your kidney, and I'm concerned that it might be a kidney cancer. So I can only imagine the anxiety with a clinical variable being relayed to a patient that has the connotations cancer does, or the connotations even the word mass does, and what kind of life changing event that conversation could be. So it's my job as the specialist expert to put that all into context for the patient. So again, orient them appropriately, give them that clinical compass that allows them to make effective decisions about their healthcare.

When I'm looking at CTs and MRIs, I'm looking for the problem. My "Where's Waldo," I'm finding Waldo, and then I'm figuring out the way to – at that point I then look at all the other impactful data from those images that I can get that would help me counsel the patient. A hernia, you know, some of the problematic issues that may make the treatment planning less than linear. And so, I mean that's what's going through my mind. So first and foremost identifying the problem, and then kind of figuring out, you know, my terminator – you've seen the Arnold Schwarzenegger where there's a knock on the door and it's, you know, the list of responses are printed out on his heads-up display. So I find the problem, my heads-up display spits out all the different ways that I can treat that, and then I look for other data in those images that might make one approach more favorable than another.

I think I walk them through my decision process, as to why I'm making the recommendations that I do, and the rationale. And again, I think imparting that information is stress relieving for them. It helps me because I'm teaching them about their problem and the things that are available. And I'm empowering them to be able to make, again, an effective decision for themselves.

Clearly high-risk patients I generally will give an overview of their disease regardless of their risk stratification. I will then discuss their risk stratification. And if they're high-risk folks, regardless of the cancer or the reason that makes them high risk, the disease process that makes them high risk, I will theoretically counsel them as to options available, but my recommendation for treatment will be to pursue symptom alleviating or potentially curative – again depending on the disease process – therapies. So a guy who's in retention, for instance, pick a non-cancer diagnosis, retention of urine, is placing himself at high risk for renal failure, repeat episodes of retention, urosepsis, things like that. He doesn't clearly have an overtly life-threatening condition, but clearly it's impacting quality of life, clearly it's impacting the viability or optimum working of other organ systems, in this case the kidneys. So that's a person I can tell you, hey, you can go along and leak urine in your diaper, that's an option. If you just want to be overflowing incontinent. It's not the greatest option, I honestly think you should pursue other symptom relief. And that would be self-intermittent catheterization if you're surgically phobic, or we should consider maybe surgical options to permanently alleviate the obstruction and allow you to begin urinating again. So I mean that's an odd example, but urology we always think of prostate cancer, kidney cancer, bladder cancer, I mean the counseling diatribe is more linear in terms of you need surgery, you need treatment, you need radiation. Whereas, you know, observational strategies now are only beginning to gain a foothold, and only for limited cancers, i.e. the small or low volume prostate cancers and low volume renal or small renal lesions. So we don't have the . . .

I think the surgery is – urologists are odd birds, because we're fairly easygoing I think as a culture, a specialty culture. But we all are somewhat Type A in that we like that instant gratification that some manipulation or intervention can give, and surgery being that intervention. So everybody likes to operate. So on the days that I operate, if you look at my – I guess if I were to wear some monitor that measured my biorhythms, I would probably be on higher biorhythms during the day I operate because I mean, you know, it's a competition, it's exciting, it's in many respects it's fun. That's why I chose urology was to have my hands – or a surrogate for my hands, my telescope and instruments – in a person, manipulate them to effect some positive change in that person. So those are fun days. Urology's also unique in that there's an element of linear care that goes on, or longitudinal care that goes on with patients. So our patients that we operate on typically have conditions that will require surveillance, unlike surgeons who – a general surgeon I mean – who may operate on somebody and see them within the first 90 days just to make sure that that person is recovering well, remove their staples, and say hey, pat on the back, go see your medical oncologist for the follow-up of your colon cancer, or go see your primary care doctor for your general health concerns because your hernia is taken care of. Urologists, if we operate on somebody typically we have that person has selected us and we've selected them for longitudinal care because that's we do our own cancer surveillance, we do our own in many cases post-operative adjuvant therapy if necessary, prostate cancer we give hormones and things like that. I think that surgery is exciting and I think that surgery offers me the opportunity, and it's kind of like an invitation to participate in that patient's care lifelong. I'm going to see them, I know, beyond three months. I'm going to see them for many years.

With the exception of bladder cancer, most of the people that we engage surgically have non – I don't want to use that term, I was going to say non-lethal. Most of our patients do well. A small percentage of gentleman with prostate cancer that we interact with, we being urologists, are going to have dissemination of their disease and demise. The majority of patients that we interact with our kidney cancers have localized T1 lesions that have an extremely high cure rates well in excess of 90 percent. Bladder cancer, not so much. Kidney stones, again, bladder outlet obstruction, again, most of those patients do well. So our linear care generally is good, and our post-operative care is much less stressful for both patient and provider than perhaps some other disciplines who have interaction, for instance a medical oncologist. If the longer you have a diagnosis of cancer the more trials of chemotherapy you go through, clearly your odds of survival start to go down. And I imagine at least for me in my mindset it would become completely depressing if I was sitting across from a patient that I knew probably had less than a 50/50 percent chance of long-term survival. I don't have that worry in urology. I think that's probably why we're reasonably easygoing people is because it's just the nature of our practice is the patients generally do pretty well.

Yeah, well, I mean it should be fun, right? I honestly I think patients do better if they have more information and I think patients do better if you can orient them in terms of their clinical compass. I keep using that term, but I honestly the difference between picking a fight with somebody whom you've really researched and you know that they always punch off their right foot so that you can expect that – I mean somebody who's better prepared has less stress, and that's both physician better prepared, patient better prepared. They should have less stress, so that when they're in that clinical environment it's not as daunting. So it should be, in some respects, fun, I guess. Yeah. It shouldn't be a problem – there are always unknowns.

And there are always patients you can't orient, do you know what I mean? Obviously they have a cognitive deficit, or perhaps they're overwhelmed with the power of the original scenario, I have cancer. And you're talking to them and you may be fluent, and you may be very effective as a speaker, but as a receptor it's just going phew right through them and they're not soaking any of it in. And those are a little bit stressful conversations. They're not fun. But you take as much time as you need. And to get it to sink in, maybe even if bringing them back.

I think for appropriately selected men, active surveillance may be the biggest impactful treatment tool that we've had in the last half decade to a decade. And it's only gained legs in probably the last five years. It's design I think is very noble. It's not, remember, active surveillance is not the engagement of a cancer with no intent to treat, that's watchful waiting. Active surveillance is to watch a cancer in an attempt to, I guess, engage it at an appropriate time, a window in which cure is available and necessary. And in doing that, we've eliminated a lot of unnecessary surgeries with a lot of unnecessary morbidity to the patient. And it's not inconsequential morbidity, I think the biggest ones we worry about are sexual function and continence. And if you have no operation, clearly you're not going to have those side effects. I mean other ones we don't even think about in the conversation are anesthetic misadventures and bleeding and injury to other organ structures or fistula. I mean these things happen, they happen at a much lower rate, but if you kind of minimize a patient's exposure to those, to the encounters that are unavoidable, you know, when it absolutely needs to be in place, I think you've done them a service. So I do advocate active surveillance for appropriately selected people.

Oh I think active surveillance has – put it this way, active surveillance has had a significant impact on the number of prostatectomies that are being performed in the treatment of prostate cancer. It's to the point that the manufacturer of the robotic system that we typically use in the performance of our surgery has completely shifted their focus away from urology and is concentrating now on gynecology and other surgical disciplines in order to gain or maintain market share and sell more products. I think urology, because of the nature of the surgery, it was a great fit for the robot initially. I think that much of the data that spun out of the surgical experience with the robot, and popularized surgical treatment for prostate cancer, rolled out on men who probably in retrospect – and this doesn't mean that the people publishing those things were bad people, just given the information and now we have a better understanding of the natural history of the disease – but a lot of that data was generated on men likely with non-lethal disease. And as a consequence, you know, it's we were exposing, in retrospect, men to overtreatment, which I think given the morbidities associated with the treatment was probably – is unacceptable. And I think we as a community, we being urology including our local community, have acknowledged that hey, we were operating on far too many men. And we need to pull back on the reins, so to speak, because we're having an impact on these gentlemen's lives that is measured not in months of recovery but in years of post-therapy convalescence. And you know, if we're operating on a fifty-five-year-old guy, that's potentially three decades of having to wear a pad, three decades of a change, significant change, in their sexual interactions with their partner. So we're on page, as a community.

There's some trepidation. I love doing the surgery, it's a great surgery, and I thank God, knock wood, our patients have excellent outcomes. But I can appreciate how it's confusing as a patient diagnosed with prostate cancer, which way they should go. And again, I think arming them with information is the greatest tool I can give them. And then the second tool I can give them is should they choose surgery, being the surgical provider for that surgery. But I think the best justice I do for my patients with prostate cancer is helping them put their cancer in perspective, and finding out where they are, the landscape of treatments in their disease.

How did you get to this place in your career?

I think urologists by and large have the same epiphany in their overall experience, we all – and I have this conversation very frequently with medical students, all get interested in urology because we've met a urologist that we liked, okay? In my instance, he was a third year urology trainee in the stairwell of the VA, in Mercury Park. And I remember vividly I was – being a third year medical student on your surgical rotation is back in oh God, this would be back in the late '80s, middle '80s, was hard work, right? They called us scut monkeys, do you remember? [laughs] And so you had all of this just like hard work, little reward, service, service, service. And I was walking after lunch or something in a stairwell, and I'll never forget it, and this guy literally jumped – he had to move from one floor to the other so fast that he wasn't even stepping on the steps but literally jumping from the top platform, holding on to the rail, down on to the next platform. And then he'd make the turn at the landing and do the same thing. So I'm hearing this jump, boom, steps, jump, boom, steps. And it's him. And he's like, "Hey, are you rotating on surgery?" And I said, "Yeah." And he goes, "What are you doing right now?" And I said, "Nothing." And he goes, "Come on with me, we're going to surgery." And we literally we went into a surgery with a guy by the name of George Hollander, who has since I think gone on and retired. He was the chairman at Syracuse for a while. And we did a nephrectomy and it was great, and the atmosphere in the room was light and nonstressful, because clearly the people involved knew what they were doing – in my naïve perspective – knew what they were doing, they clearly had a good plan, the surgery went very straightforward, and it was done. And they looked at me and they said, hey, next time we've got a case you're welcome to scrub in. So my first encounter, like many of the men and women who go into urology, my first encounter with a urologist was a tremendously positive experience, because good personality, nice surgery, very straightforward. It appealed to me. So, you know, you move on, your curiosity is piqued, you seek out those experiences more and more. And I found out that urology was a very nice blend of my instant gratification needs, tempered by my also the affinity I have for longitudinal care and experience with patients. And then my moving into urology residency was an extension of that. And then my moving into an academic career beyond urology was an extension of I like to talk. My family, my mother was an elementary school teacher, so I probably got some of her rubbing off on me. I like to teach and pass things on. So it just seems like it was a nice evolution, so to speak, of my career. It was my destiny.

Dr. Spangler's perspective

Well, I guess the first thing I do is even before that day I always try to prep for these visits so that I don't walk in blind. Nothing more disconcerting than walking in blind because then they expect you to remember stuff and know things about them, and unless it's a new patient, for example, you kind of want to have some form of plan or options for different treatment plans or follow-up plans or something. Well, usually I kind of know what those results are already, because I like to look at my own films, as you know. I like to look at the labs myself and plot them so I know how they've done in the last six months, a year, however long they've been with me. I have patients that have been with me for eight, nine years. So I don't have to go back because in my mind I already know. But it's helpful time to time to regroup with the patient as well. But I do that typically when I'm not in clinic because then if I did that in clinic I would have to think about what the plan is, and I'd like to do that beforehand so that I can expect the plan while I'm in clinic. And I think that's harder and harder to do the more patients you have, the busier you are, the more administrative and research responsibilities, so that on your off time it's hard. There have been nights where I have had to do it just by myself just to know this is what's going on, because I don't like to walk in blind to any clinical setting. Because I feel like then I haven't done my homework for that patient, and something as silly as gee is that drug covered under their plan, I want to know beforehand. Because I don't like to offer it and go, ooh, sorry about that, your Blue Cross network doesn't cover that and you're going to have to pay five grand or something godawful.

So in order to do that, much like what I've done today, is I prep with my team so that we have a variety of things already sorted out. Those variety of things could be insurance clearance, which sometimes will delay your day. And a lot of the drugs I give are high cost so they require some sort of preauthorization, which takes more than that moment. So usually it's 48 hours. The second thing is I try to put in my mind where is this person in their cancer treatment? Are they actively being treated? Are they the beginning, the middle, the end? Are they in follow-up? And that sort of changes how I view the visit. You know, if it's something that is information gathering and I'm discussing what will be the treatment plan I need to be in a different mindset than if it's more a hospice talk or end-of-life discussion. And then it's a different discussion than you're now finished with active therapy and you're in follow-up with me for five years. So with all that I kind of I put in sort of what that visit is going to be about so I don't walk in blind for that day. I already know for the, you know, twenty or thirty patients I'm going to see, these are the things that I have to talk about. And then when I'm actually there I learn to, you know, not – after you say the hello part I kind of ask one or two questions but then the majority of them already have stuff to tell me. So sometimes it's easier if I just let them tell me what it is that they want to talk about or have questions, and then I kind of go into my thing. And then we end the visit. That's usually how it goes.

It's like creating that roadmap. I think that's where patients get that sense of confidence that you have a clue as to what you're doing. So I always like to rehash, okay, why I think this is why the treatment plan is. This is your studies from the bloodwork, this is what your scans show, this is where you are in space. For example like in prostate cancer, unfortunately all these things reveal that you're now metastatic, which is totally different than when we thought everything was confined to the prostate and now these are the treatment options and why the treatment options are the way they are. Kind of go a little bit into the biology of the cancer and why the treatment is to shut down the androgen pathway. And then once I get through that kind of thinking it's a lot more clear. And then when I sort of set the expectation it's going to be, for example, oh I'm going to treat you with some hormones, but I don't leave it at that, because people don't know what that means. So I have to explain, I'm putting you into man menopause. And then all of a sudden, ding, the lightbulb goes on and they're like, oh, oh! And then chuckle, chuckle from the wife or the significant other, and then we go into that for a while, into what that means for that patient, and then they need additional therapy after that, then it's a whole 'nother discussion. So each thing takes – each step takes some discussing on a lay level so that they feel they're keeping up with me.

I would say the majority of time they follow along. There are certain cases where I do that and then they're like, oh, yeah I'm totally not going to do that. I'm not going to give up my sexual function, for example, just so I can get my PSA lower or live longer, it's not worth it. And on occasion I get that. Then we have to talk about well, these are the things that may happen. And it's not that I don't treat them anymore, we just have a different goal setting. Then we say, all right, it's within your right. I could tell you that it's not something I recommend, but I don't cast them off to the side because they don't do what I tell them to do. I just say, this is how we want to approach it. We're going to maximize your quality of life, and we'll deal with symptoms. And I'll see them periodically back. So I think it's a matter of expectation on both sides. And there are folks that come in and they're completely like, okay, I don't want anything that you're saying here, but I'm going to do completely natural therapy. And I tell them I have no data on that. But could I still be their doctor? My answer is always yes, unless it's something completely that I'm ethically not, you know, supportive of. But usually let's say it's a person that wants to do 100 percent natural therapy, I tell them this is not the way to go, but I don't want you to take a whole bunch of stuff and then your liver goes to pieces and you don't know what happened. So I'll follow them with that. And most likely after a couple months of that they revert back to, okay, you tell me what to do, because they realize that it's not working. So inevitably if I just sort of meet them halfway so that they know their expectation, they know my expectation, they know what I consider standard, not standard, then it's much more fruitful relationship, I think, on both sides, because then we know exactly what to expect from one another.

You know, I think it's tough. You know my practice is primarily GU [genitourinary] malignancies, so I get the eighteen-year-old kids, truly kids, who are almost pediatric, with testicular cancer. Those folks are probably the hardest for me. Much the reason why I didn't pick peds is because I'm perhaps too empathic to them, and I feel their pain – like I feel it. I just sort of envision if that was my child, you know, how I would feel as a parent. So knowing that's a challenge for me I have to overcome that. Keep a brighter face, try to talk to them and connect so that they follow up. Because that's a five-year follow-up. A lot of the onus is on them to do that. So a lot of the times knowing that I have to switch gears a little bit and say, okay, you know, this visit has to be more like a peds visit. It can't be scary. It can't be the visit I had with my seventy-year-old. It just has got to be a completely different thing. And when I do that, you know, I've not lost them in follow-up. I think in all the years, almost eleven years, I've only had one person completely drop out. But that's because he was a drug addict and even his mom couldn't reach him. So that one I lost. But the rest usually know when to show up, they come back like I tell them and ask them to do. So that part is sort of a visible, cognizant thing that I know myself like we have to gear up ourselves even as a team to handle those guys a little differently. I would say that's true for most of the younger ones, even adrenal cancers. We have younger women with that, and that's a tough one. They've either got toddlers at home, and that's a whole 'nother level also of trying to deal with them. I think for the most part when they're adults and a little later on in age, my first thing when I interact with them is to say I'm really sorry they have this problem. I say that to everybody. Because I think they're so used to going from doctor to doctor, or so overwhelmed with internet searches, that you forget the humanistic aspect of just I'm just sorry you're here with me right now. [laughs] Even that's usually a mind boggler and I've had people just cry even after I said that because I don't think people have sort of recognized that it's not just information gathering but it's that feeling, you know, like gosh I had a devastating diagnosis. This changes my whole life. So just an example today, young guy with prostate cancer, just diffuse. Guy in his forties, toddlers at home, and his wife is just writing things down. And I just say I'm sorry this is happening and so on, and she just broke down. I mean this is you could see just notebook of stuff, paper after paper of her going to doctor after doctor. And I just wanted to know how they were coping, because I can only imagine if that were me how I would be coping. It's tough. So that is going to be a long journey with that patient. I hope a long time because we want them to be around. But it's I think at times overwhelming for me. Especially if I try to put myself in that shoe, like oh man, if this was happening to me or my spouse how would I deal with that? And it's I would freak out. So I try to just say the things that I would want to hear my doctor say as well. And then, you know, I tell them it's a journey. I mean if you're going to stick with me, it's a journey. Some days are longer than others. And I just try to give them every assurance possible. But they know – my favorite analogy is usually it's a marathon. And that means there's no short sprints. You're just going to have to be stuck with me for all the duration. And it will be nice when we can let each other go healthy. That's the goal.

Sometimes health insurance doesn't pay for the medicine. [laughter] It is a huge bane of my existence. It really is. And I've had too many emails fired off to our administrators because I am – not upset, but worried I think about the situation. Not only do patients really have no idea what's going on with this Affordable Care Act, practitioners don't know. Because we know the medicine part of it, but we don't know truly the business and insurance part of it. Unfortunately, the drugs I prescribe, especially in prostate and kidney cancer, are in the thousands per month. So one bottle is sometimes eight, nine thousand. That's one pill, one bottle, not including their blood pressure, cholesterol, everything else they have to have, they're mostly bankrupt by the time we're done fantasizing about what great treatment plan we're going to have. So the other part of the job in prepping is that we almost have to check in advance for mostly everything. Even an injection, like (Lupron) or (Fermagon) for example, that's a high-cost item if your insurance doesn't cover it. And you assume they're going to cover it, but landscape's changed. So stuff that I've never had to worry about last year I'm worrying about this year. Secondly everyone's donut holes and deductibles are all different again. And that is a huge problem because most cancer patients rack up to that deductible within the first month or two. Well, a lot of people are coming off the holidays, they don't have that kind of cash to expend. So how do you work that? Do you hold off treatment until they have the money? No, that's silly. But it's not silly if the institution isn't getting paid. So it's this sort of up and down give or take, and I've had to change a few things based on what is covered. But that's not the same as that blood pressure medicine is covered, so is that, they're sort of similar, they're both ACE inhibitors. That's not the same, like well that prostate pill's kind of the same – no, we don't have duplicates like that. So they're not sort of interchangeable, you need to add them on as you go. That's a challenge. It's a huge problem. It's a huge problem nationwide. I hope we fix it. I don't see that going away any time soon.

I hug a lot of my outpatients because I know them well and you get sort of involved in their lives and so on. When you're an inpatient, you're the pinch hitter. You're now the doc to cover all of these folks who are obviously so gravely ill they're in the hospital. And I think in the beginning I used to have that same style. But I think it became more awkward as an inpatient because they don't know me, and those that need the hugs or the touch I will do that and I can sense that. But there are equally many patients who don't have any connection to me, and I'm just sort of the deliverer usually of bad news, sadly. And that's a tough model we have. And I don't see that improving either, because now we switched our models, which I'm not sure if you knew about that. But it's a whole different system now where we don't have residents, which makes it even more challenging, we now have hospitalists. So they – it's work in progress, let's put that out there, it's a work in progress. Yeah.

How did you get to this place in your career?

I'd like to say I got here due to a lot of guidance of other people. I don't think that I woke up one day and said, wow, I am going to be the doctor that I am. I think I'm much better than I thought that I could ever be. I think in the beginning although I'm always sort of upbeat and happy and enthusiastic, I don't think that always translates to you being a good doctor. I think with maturity I know that I'm much more patient in listening to the gripes and don't have to feel like I have to solve everything and just know that this is a relationship per se as opposed to a one-time, okay, here's your problem, I'm going to fix it and go. I think knowing that puts me a little bit more at ease to sort of just open up and say, this is what I think right now. It may change. And I'm more comfortable with that. I think when you're younger, you want to solve everything. You're going to be the fixer for everything. And I realize as I've grown older, have my own kids, that that doesn't happen all the time, and that's okay. That it's okay. That you don't have to be 100 percent every time. And so not having that kind of pressure I think, you know, sort of says look we're all human. I'm doing my best to help you right now. Maybe I'll be better another day, maybe I'll be worse another day, but I'm always going to try my absolute best for that moment. I think sort of recognizing that makes me the way I am. And I think also modeling after people that you've watched. It doesn't have to be somebody who's more senior than you, just other people that you interact with. You either know oh I don't like the way that person said that, or ooh I really like that, I'm going to take that pearl and incorporate it into something. It's part of the reasons why, for example, being in the [Gold Humanism] society it's so nice because you still learn even from students today the way they're doing their patient interaction or their stories, you're like oh that's very good, I didn't think about that. Because it's all just matter of how they feel they're helping people. So, guess that's the short answer to a very big question.

I think one of the big challenges as we move forward is sort of to retain the patient-interaction relationship in the days of the digital era, and sort of this huge new world we're encountering. Even computerizing things and social media. One of the things I'm interested in is how do you communicate with patients? If you can't just say we're using a patient portal. Again, my testicular patients will text me often. They don't talk, but they have no problem texting 2,000 paragraphs of stuff how they feel. How do you incorporate that into a note? They're not going to call you, they're not going to – that's how they communicate with each other. So I don't think if we evolve with the way technology is and be cognizant of the fact we have to maintain relationships and patient safety and patient confidentiality, medicine's not going to evolve in the right way. We have to pay attention to that.

Appendix C
Codebook and themes

The code name appears first. The number of items in the dataset using that code appears immediately after the code name. The next paragraph is an exemplar of that code from the complete dataset. The exemplars may or may not appear in the text.

Narrative Schema ($N = 97$) – Source of story components; from whom or from where. Also the construction of the story, including antecedent cultural categories used to create a narrative for the self, cultural, or social "body."

Dr. Spangler was dictating while she was looking at the previous notes so she was reading the notes and dictating relevant sections back into the computer. She was using this primarily to get the history right and then flipped to the vital signs sheet which was recorded on paper that was generated during office visit and then flipped to the labs and began reading the labs from computerized lab displayed back into her office visit note for that particular day.

Diagnosis ($N = 175$) – A mutually agreed upon label for explanation of distressing symptoms; an explanatory category.

The wife and the eldest daughter both had legal pads and were taking notes. Throughout the entire interview the patient spoke initially giving the details of dates and a diagnostic studies and scans. He actually had a parallel record typewritten in the folder that said Connaught on the cover. He was able to pull dates, results of tests out and specific treatments throughout the entire interview.

Uncertainty ($N = 65$) – Unknown, not quantifiable.

I don't want him to have to, have to sit here and tell me all kind of jokes. No, that's what I want from you, I just want you to sit down and explain everything very, very logically. Not logically; very, very easily, so I understand all these words you're using. Because if you're using some words I don't know — I can remember when my son was studying for his, one of his tests, and I was asking him questions, but I don't know what I was asking him. You know, so that's what I'm talking about. I want somebody to tell me, so I know what I'm talking about.

Social Practice ($N = 186$) – The cultural body; descriptions of who, what, where, when, and why of observed behaviors.

Most of the medical personnel labeled with badges indicating their specialty, hospital affiliation, medical school affiliation, etc., the entire labeling system for personnel is quite complex.

If a patient was to have a biopsy during clinic hours, Carmen and Dr. Jeffries could complete an entire biopsy routine wordlessly. Each anticipated the movements of the other and they coordinated the many different sequences flawlessly and efficiently. Carmen and Dr. Jeffries worked silently, not even looking in the same direction at the same time, but each completing what the other was doing. Dr. Jeffries would point to the ultrasound screen, and Carmen would move the rollerball, marking exact measurements of the size of the prostate. During the punch biopsy, the tissue specimens were collected and labeled efficiently.[1] Both gave instructions to the patient at different times without any duplication of effort.

Healing ($N = 80$) – A hypothesis code; an exploratory code to identify social practices related to the topic of interest.

The patient was very pleased. Dr. Rivers gave him a very positive prognosis and told him based on the first ten months of follow-up he doesn't expect to have any problems and he thinks will be just fine. They ended the visit with a very firm handshake and smiles all around the room. The patient left.

I had written in my scratch notes next to Dr. Smith's name: "tender caring bedside manner." I showed him what I had written and he replied, "That extra 30 seconds to a minute makes a big difference, even if you just listen. Sometimes it works, and sometimes it doesn't. You can tell the patients like it. Like the patient with the small bowel obstruction. Sometimes I go up there in the afternoon when I have nothing to do and spend five minutes just talking, but not necessarily about his medical condition. I think it helps the patient to talk to the doctor about things other than what's going on; otherwise, you don't know anything about him and nothing about the context of the patient's illness. I think it makes it better."

Disruption ($N = 91$) – Deviation from a cultural lifecourse at any level or of any type resulting in distress. I derived this code from anthropological exploration of social narratives, which were included in the data collection. I use the heuristic of ritual to organize the manuscript, which explains why all the data seems to relate to ritual. From that perspective, I selected *disruption* as a proxy for existential threats in the presentation of the data.

I was mostly concerned with ending up with a diaper. I've seen too many men my age at my complex who are either having to wear a diaper or they're dribbling or one problem after another. And I just was really concerned with that. Dr. Rivers said, "Well, what about your sex life?" I said, "At 77 years of age, I don't have a sex life." And that is hardly a thing that is important to me. What is important is the quality of life not having to wear a diaper. So I went through the procedures there; I can't remember whether it was 29 or 32 days of [treatment with] radiation every day.

Dr. Jeffries referred to the genital area as "dog meat" when he was showing the residents the extent of the injury. The anatomy is not even recognizable to the surgeon and the "repair" required to address the existential threat was to create an alternative urinary system with the suprapubic catheter and urine collection bag that replaced the urethra and bladder during this time of bodily disruption.

Emotion (N = 106) – A socially engaged cognition. Used in the way described by Keith McNeal.

I did tell Dr. Stein that he no longer scares me and Marsha said yes Dr. Stein can be quite intimidating when you first meet him. He then said something and Marsha turned around and looked at me and said, "There's hierarchy in action."

Dr. Jeffries did return and talk a little bit more about scheduling. Dr. Jeffries brought up the issue of scheduling and said, "There is no rush for surgery. You won't have any more difficulty functioning than you are now, actually less because the two weeks more of healing time." The issue of billing came up again and Dr. Jeffries reassured him again, at which time the patient became tearful.

Space (N = 66) – Cognitive apprehensions of the world; Kantian argument of reality. This is consistent with Tomasello who states, "All mammals live in basically the same sensory-motor world of permanent objects arrayed in a representational space" (1999: 16).

There's a window to the radiation room that could be seen on the computers in the control room. There's also an intercom and double video screens you can watch the patient from two different angles and talk to the patient. In the control room, as I said, up in the top left were double videos so you can always watch was going on inside. Then there were five flat-panel computer screens all lined up. The one on the far left had three fields displayed. The middle one was ticking as the dose was administered. The next one had the outline of the perimeter plan.

Dr. Stein said to the patient, "We looked at the CT scan. The kidney is this big," he indicated by showing the size with his hands. "We can show you [on the computer screen]." But then he started drawing it and said, "This is the shape of your kidney, and down here there's a solid mass. Usually this is kidney cancer, and the treatment is surgical removal. If there's no spread, you can consider this a cure."

Persuasion (N = 59) – Rhetorical powers, as defined by Mattingly (1988: 5).

Also during that visit Dr. Jeffries said specifically, "Here's the story. We checked with the emergency department and they took the sample out of the bag," indicating the bag attached to this suprapubic.[2] He said, "That's always contaminated. They might as well take it and swab the floor and then send that for culture." He did this entire thing, demonstrated by putting his index finger in his mouth, dragging his index finger just above the floor surface, and making the motion of putting it into a container and sending off. He said, "If any doctors or primary contact care doctors wanted to bitch, then just drop my name and tell them they should contact me." The patient's daughter said thank you.

Dr. Stein then asked the patient to come out from the exam room and brought them over the computer and pointed to the kidney stone on the CT scan and said to the patient, "This is where the kidney stone is, right between the bladder and prostate."

Clinical Gaze – As defined by Foucault (1973; 1994).

Dr. Fields then said that he has had the experience of poor quality CT scans with Hopewell hospital. The presenter said that when he was there they were using a four head CT scanner and of course now they're using a 64 head CT scanner for most things and sometimes a 128 head. They agreed that if there was a question to simply repeat the CT scan with a higher resolution.

Dr. Stein then resumed clinical work by reviewing a CT scan image. He addressed the medical student, "The CT is easiest for me because I have more familiarity with it." He did look at the cyst on the kidney and said, "That looks benign.[3,4] It is eccentropic[5] on the left." As he was changing the slices on the CT image using the rollerball on the mouse, he pointed to and touched the screen, saying, "That is the kidney. There is a stone . . . another stone."

Computers (N = 163) – An essential tool used by healthcare personnel.

Scanned into the computer were radiation oncology records from China, all written in Chinese. Nobody knew how to read Chinese. Dr. Rivers said they were able to tell what dose to what area, which is the only information they needed. When I looked back, Dr. Rivers was sitting looking at flat-panel computer screen with his head leaning in toward the screen so the center of gravity of his head was in front of the center of gravity of his body and his hand was on the mouse. This is a typical stance of any teenager who does gaming, and I've seen it multiple times in my fieldwork. He then went on to email, and is very astute with keyboard, but they were emailing back and forth about next steps in planning radiation therapy, and so forth.

On a different occasion, I walked into the clinic and it was immediately apparent that Carmen and Dr. Jeffries were having trouble accessing clinical data. Dr. Jeffries asked Carmen, "Have we asked if they could print it and fax it, because we can't do a thing until I get them?" The administrator was talking to someone downtown in administration, simultaneously, in recognition that the difficulty accessing the information would disrupt the entire clinic schedule and cause patient dissatisfaction.

Hierarchy (N = 164) – Necessary for functionality; has the potential for abuse of power.

At one point Dr. Jeffries said that that's why he's so smart. He understands all the statistical data. Dr. Stein also pointed out that this particular trial was drug A versus drug B and that there was no placebo arm, so the size effect would be larger if there was. He said in general we believe the study. Dr.

Jeffries commented about him being smart. "That's why he's speaking in [foreign country] in front of (the prime minister) of [foreign country]."

Once we were outside the room and back the hallway, Dr. Fields said to Dr. Pinder, "This is the first time in my entire residency that I've been late; it's been 14 months and this is the first time. You showed up two minutes before I did." Dr. Pinder said, "It doesn't matter what time I show up." Dr. Fields replied, "I was hoping you wouldn't chew me out on rounds."

Positionality (N = 101) – Recognition of the duality of anthropologist – doctor and its effect on data collection.

I asked what type of patients they saw and Marsha said incontinence, cancer, bladder, renal, kidney, erectile dysfunction, BPH. She then went and gave me a list of diagnoses and highlighted the diagnoses on the billing sheet. Observer's reflection: I asked the types of patients – it could've been little old ladies, kids, or guys with prostate problems, but instead she gave me a list of diagnoses. This is now a recurrent finding: the medical assistants think of the patient's as diagnoses, the patient's pick up the language and use the language of diagnoses, and the doctors are using medical diagnoses.

I told Dr. Jeffries, "I shouldn't do this, but even without seeing the patient and only listening to you, I can almost diagnose her using the DSM-IV-R [psychiatric manual]. From a doctor to another doctor, you need to set boundaries, limit the patient's time, and if she's offended she'll go somewhere else and just consider you to be a jerk. She probably has an Axis II diagnosis,"[6] and he agreed to that. After this brief interlude I said, "I'm going to have to try and go back and be a scientist now," signaling that I was going back into observation mode.

Manuscript (N = 53) – Moments during fieldwork when event was of such important that it would be included in the dissertation manuscript as significant result.

The patient said directly to Dr. Rivers, "I'd come for you . . . You know that." She then turned, looking at me, and said, "I'm speaking for his benefit." She was referring to me. . . . There was some talk about our different roles, etc., and then after Dr. Rivers left. She asked me why I wanted to interview her, and I said, "It's because of that comment you made about him," how important it was to point out that she would do anything for Dr. Rivers. I said that's what I was interested in and then she said, "He relaxes me. I wasn't relaxed this morning, but now I am." Observer's reflection: Again I'm going to call this the "hug equivalent," because this closeness occurred after all the radiation planning, after the counseling, after the treatment, and the simple follow-up exam. There's obvious affection between the two of them, and the hug equivalent is because I heard it with Dr. Jeffries and I heard it with Dr. Spangler.

Dr. Stein then asked the patient to come out from the exam room and brought them over the computer and pointed to the kidney stone on the CT scan and said to the patient, "This is where the kidney stone is, right between the bladder and prostate."

Notes

1   A punch biopsy uses a hollow needle which is thrust into the organ to yield a core of tissue that is removed for microscopic examination.

2   Shorthand for suprapubic catheter – a tube placed through the skin above the pubic bone and inserted directly into the bladder to drain urine.

3   A cyst is a mass that is filled with fluid as opposed to solid; the significance is that cysts are very rarely malignant.

4   Benign means not malignant – cancer is only one type of malignancy.

5   This word means that the mass is growing outward from the contour of the kidney.

6   Axis II is part of a formal psychiatric diagnosis. It is not a disorder of the emotions and not a disorder of thinking – it is a personality disorder.

Index